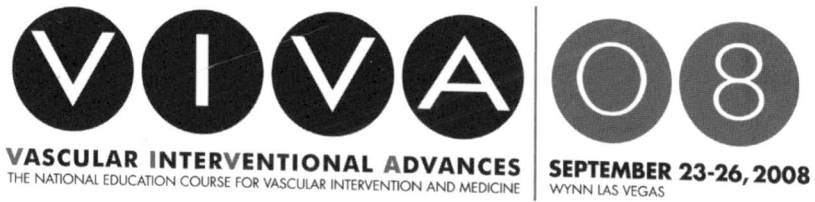

VASCULAR INTERVENTIONAL ADVANCES | **SEPTEMBER 23-26, 2008**
THE NATIONAL EDUCATION COURSE FOR VASCULAR INTERVENTION AND MEDICINE | WYNN LAS VEGAS

September 22, 2008

D1097940

Dear VIVA attendee:

Thank you for joining us at the beautiful Wynn Hotel and Casino for VIVA 2008! We hope you find the symposium intellectually stimulating and fulfilling.

Since the main mission of VIVA Physicians is education of our colleagues, we offer you this complimentary copy of "Peripheral Arterial Disease" published by the American College of Physicians. The VIVA Physicians purchased these copies as our commitment to education. We hope you find this a useful addition to your professional library.

THE VIVA COURSE DIRECTORS

This book has been purchased
with a grant provided by
St. Jude Medical.

Peripheral
Arterial
Disease

Edited by

Emile R. Mohler III, MD, FACP

Director of Vascular Medicine
University of Pennsylvania Health System
Associate Professor of Medicine
University of Pennsylvania School of Medicine
Philadelphia, Pennsylvania

Michael R. Jaff, DO, FACP

Director of Vascular Medicine
Massachusetts General Hospital
Assistant Professor of Medicine
Harvard Medical School
Boston, Massachusetts

AMERICAN COLLEGE OF PHYSICIANS

PHILADELPHIA

Associate Publisher and Manager, Books Publishing, Tom Hartman
Developmental Editor, Marla Sussman
Production Supervisor, Allan S. Kleinberg
Senior Editor, Karen C. Nolan
Editorial Coordinator, Angela Gabella
Marketing Associate, Caroline Hawkins
Cover and Interior Design, Kate Nicols
Indexer, Kathy Patterson

Manufactured in the United States of America
Printing/binding by McNaughton & Gunn
Composition by ATLIS Graphics, Gettysburg, Pennsylvania

ISBN: 978-1-930513-96-9

08 09 10 11 12 / 10 9 8 7 6 5 4 3 2 1

Dedication

To our families for their patience and support of this endeavor, and to our patients, for whom we continue to strive for better lives.

EMILE MOHLER III
MICHAEL R. JAFF

Contributors

Oliver Aalami, MD
Vascular Fellow
Northwestern University
  School of Medicine
Chicago, Illinois

Olujimi A. Ajijola, MD
Internal Medicine Resident
Massachusetts General Hospital
Boston, Massachusetts

Salman Arain, MD
Department of Cardiology
Ochsner Clinic Foundation
New Orleans, Louisiana

**Yung-Wei Chi, DO, RVT, RPVI,
  FSVMB**
Vascular Medicine Specialist
Ochsner Clinic Foundation
New Orleans, Louisiana

**F. Gerald R. Fowkes, PhD,
  FRCPE, FFPHM**
Professor of Epidemiology
University of Edinburgh
Edinburgh, Scotland

Corey K. Goldman, MD, PhD
Director of Vascular Medicine
Ochsner Clinic Foundation
New Orleans, Louisiana

Michael R. Jaff, DO, FACP
Director of Vascular Medicine
Massachusetts General Hospital
Assistant Professor of Medicine
Harvard Medical School
Boston, Massachusetts

Jon S. Matsumura, MD
Associate Professor of Surgery
Feinberg School of Medicine
Northwestern University
Chicago, Illinois

Emile R. Mohler III, MD, FACP
Director of Vascular Medicine
University of Pennsylvania Health
  System
Associate Professor of Medicine
University of Pennsylvania School
  of Medicine
Philadelphia, Pennsylvania

Thom W. Rooke, MD
Head, Section of Vascular Medicine
Mayo Clinic
Rochester, Minnesota

Wendy S. Tzou, MD
Division of Cardiovascular
  Medicine
University of Pennsylvania
Philadelphia, Pennsylvania

Ioanna Tzoulaki, MSc, PhD
University of Edinburgh
Public Health Sciences
Edinburgh, Scotland

Christopher J. White, MD
Chairman, Cardiovascular Medicine
Ochsner Clinic Foundation
New Orleans, Louisiana

Preface

Peripheral arterial disease (PAD) remains underrecognized, and the impact of this disorder on quality of life and survival is not appreciated by many health care providers. The treatment of PAD continues to evolve but is fundamentally focused on improvement in exercise performance and control of risk factors in order to prevent the associated risk of heart attack and stroke and premature cardiovascular death. The pathophysiology of progressive atherosclerotic plaque is thought to involve plaque hemorrhage and rupture, but few data support this presumption. Furthermore, there are few studies prospectively evaluating agents to halt progression of atherosclerotic disease in the lower-extremity arterial system. Despite these current limitations in understanding and treating PAD, significant strides have been made towards treatment of risk factors and strategies to improve pain-free walking distance, including the use of emerging endovascular strategies.

The primary objective of *Peripheral Arterial Disease* is to provide the reader with the most current information on diagnosis and treatment of PAD. The text is unique in that chapters are prefaced with practical and commonly asked questions regarding the diagnosis and treatment of this debilitating condition. A chapter reviewing investigative strategies, including peripheral angiogenesis, is included to provide a view of potential future therapy. Additionally, an interactive Web site is available through the American College of Physicians, which includes detailed references and continued medical education for this topic.

We hope that this reference provides an easy-to-use resource for the practicing clinician, ultimately resulting in better care for our patients.

Emile Mohler III, MD, FACP
Michael R. Jaff, DO, FACP

Contents

Visit http://www.acponline.org/peripheralarterialdisease
for additional information.

Chapter 1

Epidemiology of Peripheral Arterial Disease

IOANNA TZOULAKI, MSc, PhD
F. GERALD R. FOWKES, MBChB, PhD

1. What is the incidence/prevalence of PAD?
2. What is the natural history of PAD?
3. What risk factors increase the likelihood of limb loss?

This chapter describes the epidemiology of peripheral arterial disease (PAD). The prevalence and incidence of the disease, along with its natural history as evaluated in epidemiologic research are discussed. Finally, the established risk factors for the development and progression of PAD are summarized.

Definition of Peripheral Arterial Disease

The term "peripheral arterial disease" is widely used to refer to atherosclerotic disease that obstructs the blood supply to the lower limbs. Considerable confusion exists concerning this term because some investigators include carotid, mesenteric, renal, and upper extremity disease in the definition of PAD. The term "peripheral vascular disease" (PVD) has less specificity because, for many researchers, PVD includes venous as well as arterial disease. Other terms have been used, such as "peripheral arterial occlusive disease" (PAOD), "arteriosclerosis obliterans" (ASO), and "lower extremity arterial disease" (LEAD). Here, PAD is used solely to describe atherosclerotic disease in the arteries of the legs.

PAD starts for many individuals early in life and remains asymptomatic for a long time. It often has clinical symptoms when it is relatively advanced. The most common symptom is intermittent claudication (IC), a cramping pain in the legs that is induced by exercise and relieved by rest. When PAD progresses to severe impairment of blood flow to the limb due to arterial stenosis and occlusion, an individual is considered to have critical limb ischemia (CLI). CLI is often characterized by persistent rest pain, which becomes worse when the legs are elevated, for example in bed at night. People diagnosed with CLI may also present with gangrene and ulceration in their legs.

Prevalence and Incidence of Peripheral Arterial Disease

PAD is a relatively common condition that affects many adults worldwide (1). The prevalence (frequency at a defined time) and incidence (development of new cases) of PAD in populations has been measured in several epidemiological studies. These studies have used various definitions of PAD. Some use IC to define PAD, whereas others employ noninvasive tests such as an abnormal ankle brachial index (ABI) to measure asymptomatic forms of PAD. Few reports focus on the later disease stages of CLI, including rest pain, ulceration, or gangrene. In general, the prevalence of lower-extremity PAD varies with the age of the cohort studied, the risk-factor profile of the cohort, and the diagnostic test used to measure the disease. An overview of population studies on the prevalence and incidence of lower-extremity atherosclerosis is given here.

Intermittent Claudication

IC as a symptomatic expression of PAD defines a subset of the total population with the disease. Epidemiological studies have assessed the prevalence of IC mainly by means of the World Health Organization (WHO)/IC questionnaire (Table 1-1). Overall, the estimated prevalence of claudication assessed by an IC questionnaire ranges from 0.4% to 14.4% (2). In one of these cohorts, among 467 men and 1444 women of a hospital-based geriatrics practice, the prevalence of IC was as high as 20% in males and 13% in females (3). However, in more than 18,000 younger individuals (40-69 years old) of the UK Whitehall study, the prevalence of IC was estimated at 1.8% (4).

Some evidence that IC is slightly more common in males than in females is also presented. However, gender differences have not been observed in some studies. In the Edinburgh Artery Study of people aged 55-74 years, the prevalence of IC was the same (4.6%) in men and women (5). In support of these findings, Reunanen et al (3) reported a 2.1% prevalence in

Table 1-1.   Prevalence of Intermittent Claudication (IC) in Different Population Studies Assessed by Means of the WHO/IC Questionnaire

Reference	N	Population	Location	Age (yrs)	IC (%)
Bothig et al 1976 (72)	—	M	Moscow	50-64	6.9
		M	Berlin	50-64	3.4
Hughson et al 1978 (73)	162	MF	England	45-69	2.2
Schroll & Munck 1981 (74)	666	MF	Denmark	>60	1.8
Reunanen et al 1982 (3)	5738	M	Finland	30-59	2.1
	5224	F		30-59	1.8
Criqui et al 1985 (13)	613	MF	USA	38-82	2.2
Gofin et al 1987 (75)	1036	M	Jerusalem	40-60	1.3
	556	F			1.8
Smith et al 1990 (4)	18,388	MF	Scotland	40-64	1.8
Stoffers et al 1990 (11)	3654	MF	Holland	45-54	0.6
				55-64	2.5
				65-74	8.8
Fowkes et al 1995 (5)	1592	MF	Scotland	55–74	4.6
Dewhurst et al 1991 (76)	259	MF	England	65-95	5
Newman et al 1993 (34)	2214	M	USA	65-85	2.0
	2870	M			
Mittelmark et al 1990 (77)	5201	M	USA	>65	3.0
Arnow et al 1994 (59)	1160	M		80	32
	2464	F		81	6
Bowlin et al 1994 (78)	10,059	M	Israel	40-65	2.7
Bainton 1994 (79)	2055	M	Scotland	60-64	2.9
Wilt 1996 (80)	4159	MF	USA	—	8.5
Zheng et al 1997 (85)	1553	M†	USA	45-64	0.6
	2518	F†			0.5
	5207	M‡	USA	45-64	1.1
	5828	F‡			0.6
Meijer et al 1998 (25)	7715	MF	Holland	>55	1.6
Ness et al 2000 (81)	467	M	USA	80	20
	1444	F		81	13
Murabito et al 2002 (82)	1554	M	USA	>40	3.9
	1759	F			3.3
Brevetti et al 2004 (83)	4352	MF	Italy	40-80	1.6
Diehm 2004 (84)	6821	MF	Germany	>65	2.8

M: males, F: females
†African-American, ‡White

men and a 1.8% prevalence in women; the age-adjusted prevalence was almost equal. These findings are in keeping with an equilibration in the frequency of cardiovascular disease between men and women at older ages.

There are fewer reports on the incidence of PAD in populations. In the Framingham Heart Study, incidence of PAD was based on IC symptoms in 2336 men and 2873 women aged 29-62 years. The annual incidence was estimated to be 6 per 10,000 men and 3 per 10,000 women for those aged 30-44 years; 61 per 10,000 men and 54 per 10,000 women for those aged 65-74 years (6). On the other hand, the Quebec Cardiovascular Study (7) estimated the incidence of PAD at 41 per 10,000 population per year. In the Edinburgh Artery Study of 1529 subjects aged 55-74 years after 17 years of follow-up, 12.1% of the baseline population had experienced IC. These results demonstrate that, like the prevalence, the incidence of PAD in populations varies greatly depending on the age structure and characteristics of the population, as well as the epidemiologic methods used. However, most studies show that the incidence of PAD increases substantially with age.

Asymptomatic Disease

The prevalence of asymptomatic disease can only be estimated by noninvasive diagnostic techniques. Therefore, the estimated prevalence is greatly dependent on the actual measurement technique used in each study. The ratio of the ankle to the brachial systolic pressure, called the "ankle-brachial index" (ABI), the "ankle-brachial pressure index" (ABPI), or the "ankle-arm index" (AAI), is the cornerstone of noninvasive assessment of patients with symptomatic or asymptomatic PAD. The normal ABI should be greater than or equal to 1. An ABI less than unity (or less than 0.9 in practice) at rest indicates hemodynamically significant arterial obstruction in the legs (8). Like many biological variables, the distribution of ABI in the general population is bell shaped. However, with the ABI there are relatively more subjects having lower levels, probably due to the occurrence of atherosclerotic disease (Figure 1-1). Other noninvasive tests include pulse palpation, flow velocity determination, and duplex ultrasound.

In general, the prevalence of asymptomatic disease is higher than that estimated on the basis of IC symptoms and ranges between 0.9% and 22%, with the ratio of symptomatic to asymptomatic ranging between 1:0.9 and 1:6.0 (9). Pioneer research by Hiatt et al (10) showed that for every individual with IC there are another three with asymptomatic disease causing a 50% or greater stenosis of the arteries supplying the legs. The predominance of asymptomatic patients was also demonstrated by Stoffers (11), who investigated the prevalence of asymptomatic PAD in a population of 18,884 people aged 45-74 years and found that, although the disease was diagnosed in 6.9% by an ABI <0.95, only 22% of these people had symptoms of PAD.

The BASLE Study 12 in 1959 was among the first studies to measure the prevalence of asymptomatic disease using pulse waveforms detected on os-

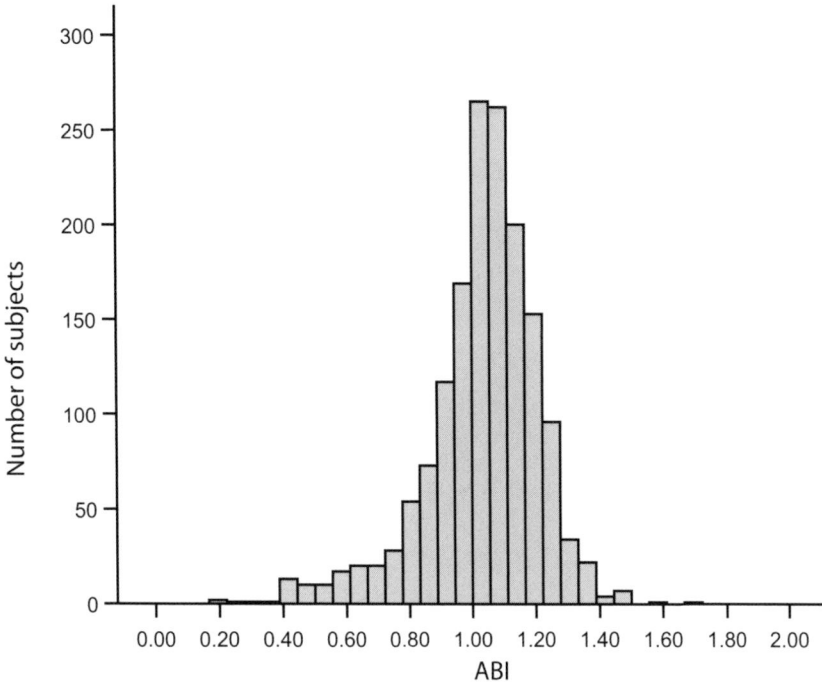

Figure 1-1.   Distribution of the minimum ankle brachial index (ABI) of the left or right leg in 1,592 subjects in the general population in the Edinburgh Artery Study.

cillography. Among men the prevalence of occlusion confirmed by arteri-ography was 7.5% in those aged 60-64 years. Later, Criqui et al (13) used three different diagnostic tests (ABI, pulse wave analysis, and pulse exam-ination) along with the WHO questionnaire in 613 men and women in California to define PAD. The prevalence of PAD was 12%, which was con-siderably higher than that estimated by the claudication questionnaire alone (2.2%).

The vast majority of epidemiological studies use the ABI >0.9 alone to define asymptomatic PAD. Although there is not a valid cut-off point to de-fine PAD, this ABI level is thought to correlate well with the severity of dis-ease across different populations. Among 2174 individuals older than 40 years participating in the US National Health and Nutrition Examination Survey (14), 4.3% had an abnormal ABI (<0.9). Recently, the PAD Awareness, Risk and Treatment (PARTNERS) Study (15) measured the ABI in 6979 primary care patients aged 70 years or older or aged 50-69 years with a history of smoking or diabetes. The PARTNERS program focused on subjects at increased risk rather than the general population or a healthy group and found that PAD defined as ABI <0.9 was present in 29% of the study population. This study provided further evidence that differences in prevalence of PAD between genders are very small; the prevalence of PAD in women was almost identical to that in men, despite the fact that other cardiovascular disease was almost twice as common in men as in women.

The incidence of asymptomatic disease shows similar age and sex patterns as prevalence but has been studied less frequently. For example, in 2327 Dutch subjects, after 7.2 years the overall incidence rate for asymptomatic PAD, assessed with ABI <0.9, was 9.9 per 1000 person-years at risk (16). In this cohort, it was also noted that the incidence of asymptomatic PAD was higher than the incidence of symptomatic PAD, with women developing PAD more often than men.

Critical Limb Ischemia

There is little information on the incidence and prevalence of CLI. It has been estimated in the UK that there are approximately 20,000 people with CLI in the population, with an annual incidence of 400 per million per year (17). Catalano et al (18) calculated the incidence of CLI using different approaches in an Italian population. A 7-year follow-up of 200 people with IC and 180 controls indicated that the incidence of CLI was 450 per million per year. Alternatively, looking at the hospitalizations for CLI for a sample of hospitals, the incidence of CLI was 652 per million per year. Recently, the Oxford Vascular Study (19) followed up 19,106 subjects to record noncoronary event rates. After 3 years, the rate for CLI was 0.34 per 1000 population per year and 0.38 and 0.29 in males and females, respectively.

On the assumption that all amputations are performed for CLI and that 25% of people with CLI require amputation, the incidence of CLI can be estimated between 500-1000 per million per year (9). Another approach would be to look at the prevalence of IC and assume that 5% of claudicants will progress to CLI after 5 years. Then the incidence of CLI is approximately 300 per million per year, and approximately one patient per year will develop CLI for every 100 with IC (9).

Recently, Jensen et al (20) used a questionnaire to estimate the prevalence of CLI in 20,291 Norwegian men and women aged 40-69 years. The authors defined CLI as ulcer in the toes, foot, or ankle that have failed to heal and/or persistent pain in the forefoot while in supine position with relief of the pain when standing up (20). They found that the prevalence of CLI was 0.26% among men and 0.24% among women.

Risk Factors for Developing Peripheral Arterial Disease

Specific risk factors have been associated with the development and progression of peripheral atherosclerosis. Figure 1-2 shows the range of relative risks for some important factors defined in epidemiological studies published by the Trans-Atlantic Inter-Society Consensus (TASC) Working Group on the management of peripheral arterial disease (9).

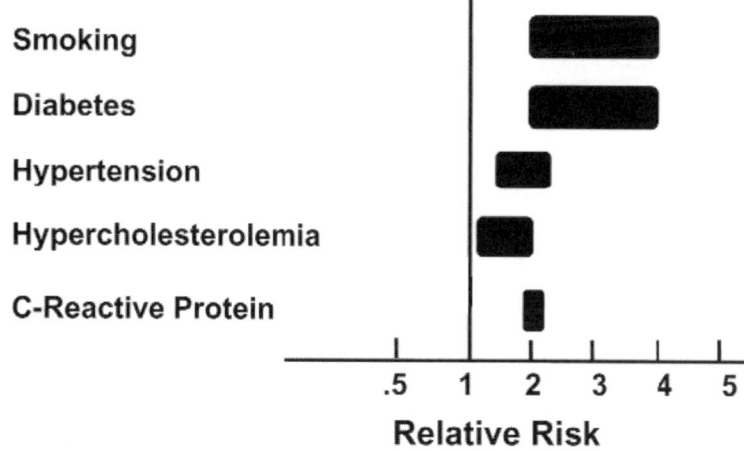

Figure 1-2. Risk of developing lower extremity PAD. The range for each risk factor is estimated from epidemiological studies. The relative risks are estimated for current vs. ex smokers and nonsmokers, presence vs. absence of diabetes and hypertension, and top vs. bottom quartile of C-reactive protein. The estimate for hypercholesterolemia is based on a 10% risk for each 10 mg per dL rise in total cholesterol. Adapted with permission from Dormandy JA, Rutherford RB. Management of peripheral arterial disease (PAD). TASC Working Group. TransAtlantic Inter- Society Consensus (TASC). J Vasc Surg 2000;31(1 pt 2):S1-S296.

Overall, epidemiological studies have shown that risk factors for PAD are almost identical to those associated with coronary heart disease (CHD). However, some, such as smoking, would appear to be particularly important in the development of peripheral atherosclerosis. The importance of age and sex was already mentioned in the previous section, which showed that prevalence and incidence of PAD increased with age and was slightly more common in males than females. Here, a brief review of epidemiologic data on well-established risk factors for the development of PAD is given.

Smoking

All epidemiological studies have confirmed that smoking is a strong risk factor for PAD. In the Framingham study, 78% of patients with IC were smokers (21), whereas in the Edinburgh Artery Study the risk of developing the disease was 3-fold higher in smokers than in non-smokers (22). Data from these two studies also showed that diagnosis of PAD was made almost a decade earlier than in non-smokers. A recent meta-analysis of 4 prospective and 13 cross-sectional studies reported that the overall prevalence of symptomatic PAD was increased 2.6-fold in current smokers and 2.3-fold in ex-smokers (23). The importance of smoking in PAD has been shown to be stronger than in coronary artery disease (CAD). In the Framingham Study the risk in smokers compared with non-smokers for

PAD was double compared with the risk for CAD (21). A clear dose-response relationship with a strong increase in risk for PAD in heavy smokers has also been reported.

Diabetes Mellitus

Overall, epidemiological evidence confirms an approximately 2- to 4-fold increase in prevalence of PAD in people with diabetes compared with those without it (21,22). In studies using the ABI, the prevalence of PAD (defined as an ABI <0.90) in diabetic individuals ranges from 20% to 30% (15,24). Moreover, data from the Framingham and Rotterdam studies have shown increased rates of absent pedal pulses, femoral bruits, and decreased ABI in people with diabetes (25,26). The duration and severity of diabetes would appear to correlate with the incidence and extent of PAD (27).

Diabetic peripheral arterial disease often affects distal limb vessels, such as the tibial and peroneal arteries, limiting the potential for collateral vessel development (28). As a result, patients with diabetes are more likely to develop severe symptomatic forms of the disease such as rest pain or ulceration as well as IC (27). In the Framingham study for both sexes, diabetes was associated with a 2- to 3-fold excess risk of IC compared with its absence (29).

Blood Lipids

The effect of blood lipids on PAD is less clear. It has been suggested that the association between elevated cholesterol levels and PAD seems to be somewhat weaker than that for CHD. In the Framingham study, people with IC had a higher mean cholesterol level; people with total cholesterol >270 mg/dL had twice the incidence of developing IC (6). Similarly in the NHANES study (14), 2174 subjects older than 40 years with a total cholesterol of 240 mg/dL or greater had a risk ratio of 1.88 for PAD defined by ABI <0.9. Interestingly, these results were not replicated by other studies (30).

Similar evidence was found for decreased HDL levels. In the Rotterdam study, total cholesterol, but not HDL cholesterol, was associated with an ABI <0.9 (25). However, in the Edinburgh Artery Study, both increased total and decreased HDL cholesterol were independently associated with IC and with ABI <0.9 (22). Ridker et al (12) compared LDL, HDL, triglycerides, and ratio of total/HDL cholesterol as predictors of PAD and found the latter to have the greatest independent effect. Evidence that treatment of hyperlipidemia reduces both the progression and the incidence of PAD has also been found (32). Finally, an association between increased triglycerides and PAD has been reported by many studies, but the strength of this association is reduced on multivariate analysis, and the effect of triglycerides on PAD remains unclear (2,30).

Hypertension

Epidemiologic studies have confirmed an association between increased blood pressure levels and PAD, and they estimated that approximately 50%-92% of claudicants have hypertension (33). In the US Cardiovascular Health Study, 52% of patients with asymptomatic PAD (ABI ≤0.9) had high blood pressure; hypertension was associated with the progression of PAD, defined by declining ABI after 6 years of follow-up (34,35). Follow-up data from the Framingham Study demonstrated a 2.5- to 4-fold increased risk of developing IC in men and women with hypertension (6). In the Golstrup study, significant correlations were found between initial elevated systolic and diastolic blood pressure and ABI after 10 years (3). This was also suggested in the Edinburgh (22) study, although not by the Whitehall study (4), which found no association between hypertension and PAD. Overall, high blood pressure is likely to be a risk factor for PAD but may not be as important as other risk factors, such as smoking (Figure 1-3).

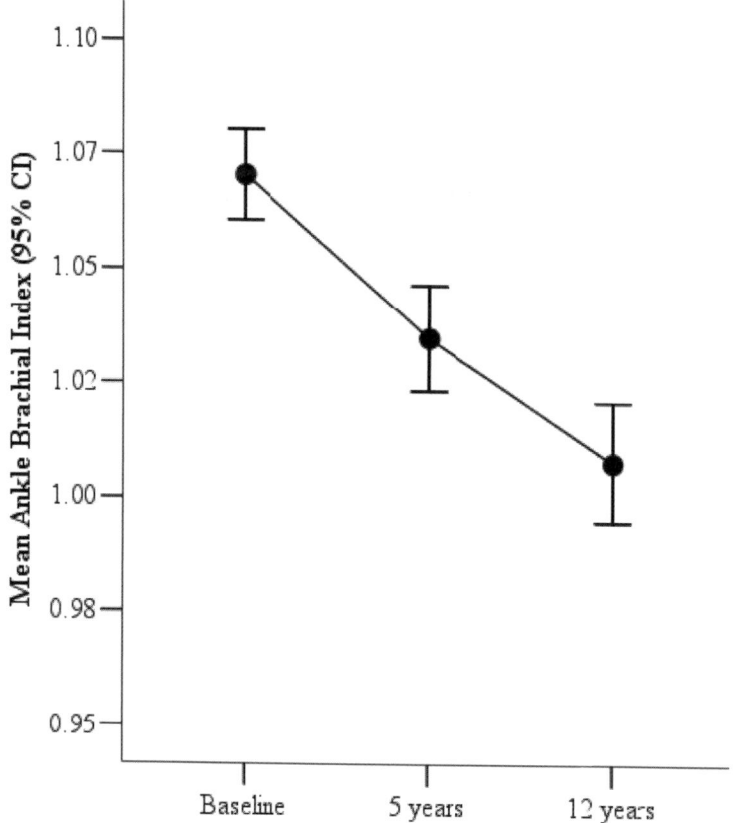

Figure 1-3.   Mean ankle brachial index (ABI) (95% CI) of the 754 subjects who had measures of ABI at baseline, 5 and 12 years examination in the Edinburgh Artery Study.

Inflammatory and Hemostatic Factors

With advances in molecular biology, a series of plasma markers reflecting activated inflammation and hemostasis have been proposed as potential risk factors for atherosclerotic disease. Although these risk factors have been mainly studied in relation to coronary or cerebrovascular disease, evidence for associations with the development of PAD exists. In a prospective study, Ridker et al (31) showed that C-reactive protein (CRP), an acute phase reactant, was associated with a 2-fold increase in the risk for future PAD, independent of conventional risk factors. Associations between another phase reactant, fibrinogen, with PAD has also been observed in the Edinburgh Artery Study and the US Physicians' Health Study (31,36).

Fewer data exist in relation to vascular adhesion molecules, such as intercellular adhesion molecule-1 (ICAM-1) and soluble adhesion molecule-1 (VCAM-1). ICAM-1, and not VCAM-1, has been associated with a more than 3-fold increase in the risk of developing symptomatic PAD in analysis adjusted for cardiovascular disease risk factors (37). IL-6 has also been associated with decline in ABI during 12 years of follow-up, independent of cardiovascular risk factor and other inflammatory markers, in the Edinburgh Artery Study (38). Fibrinolytic factors such as D-dimer and t-PA have also shown associations with incident PAD (36).

Despite the aforementioned evidence, the role of these plasma markers in peripheral and systemic atherosclerosis is not well-established and awaits to be confirmed from further epidemiological and clinical research.

Other Risk Factors

Obesity and low physical activity have shown strong associations with CHD, but their relationship with PAD is not well established. Few studies have examined the relationship between obesity, mainly measured by the body mass index (BMI), and incident PAD; the overall evidence for an association was weak (16,30). As in CHD, an alternative measure of body fat, such as waist circumference or waist-to-hip ratio, might show stronger associations with incident PAD, but currently there are no data on this relationship. On the other hand, a physically active lifestyle has been associated with a reduced risk of developing PAD (39,40). However, physical activity may be particularly difficult to study in PAD because symptomatic disease may result in reduced physical activity.

Some evidence for ethnic differences in the prevalence of PAD also exists. In the San Diego population study, black ethnicity was an independent risk factor for PAD at a magnitude similar to that of other established risk factors (41). Likewise, the National Health and Nutrition Examination Survey found an increase in the risk of PAD among non-

Hispanic black individuals (14), a result that has been shown by others (34,42). The excess prevalence of PAD in blacks could not be explained by an excess of diabetes, hypertension, or other cardiovascular disease risk factors, or by any greater susceptibility to cardiovascular disease risk factors.

Progression of Local Disease in the Legs

Atherosclerotic disease of the lower extremities can progress locally (in the legs) and may also lead to systemic manifestations of the disease such as CHD or stroke. Interestingly, most people seem to experience other cardiovascular events, and fewer have worsening PAD. The progression of the latter group is described here.

Intermittent Claudication and Asymptomatic Disease

Intermittent claudication can progress in different ways, such improvement or stabilization or worsening of claudication, which may then require surgical intervention and, finally, amputation. Studies have shown that the majority of patients either improve or stabilize (9). This can be clearly seen in a review of 10 trials of patients with IC in which 75% of claudicants experienced stabilization of their symptoms over 5-18 years (43). In the Framingham Study, only about 30% of patients with IC had persistent symptoms for a minimum of 4 years (44). Additionally, symptoms progressed in only about 15%-30% of claudicants and, in total, 25% required surgery or experienced tissue loss. Finally, less than 4% of claudicants required a major amputation (45).

The rate of progression of asymptomatic disease is unclear. The data available indicate a relatively benign course as far as the legs are concerned. In the Basle study, only 20% of people with asymptomatic PAD developed IC and 8% critical limb ischemia over 10 years (46). Progression of asymptomatic disease can also be measured via noninvasive modalities such as the ABI over time. In the Edinburgh Artery Study, changes in ABI for each leg were recorded from baseline in 1988 until subsequent 5-year and 12-year clinical examinations. Figure 1-3 shows the mean ABI (lower of either leg) at three time points in 754 subjects who had measures of ABI at all time points. Interestingly, the mean ABI in the worse leg (leg with lower ABI at baseline) of study subjects showed little progression over 12 years. The decline in ABI occurred more rapidly in the limb with a higher ABI at baseline, which may indicate a systemic tendency to atherosclerosis. In the same study, individuals with IC experienced a greater decline in both legs compared with those without claudication (47).

Critical Limb Ischemia

It is particularly difficult to describe the natural history of the ischemic limb because most patients undergo some form of vascular intervention (9). The primary amputation rate ranges between 10% and 40%, whereas the remaining patients have general supportive or medical treatment. Limb loss in patients with CLI is more common than in claudicants, and 10%-40% of people with CLI need amputation (2). Results from one multicenter study showed that 61% of patients with CLI had attempted revascularization and 7% a primary amputation after 1 year of follow-up (48). In another multicenter study, 44.4% of patients with CLI had attempted revascularization and 9.4% amputation after 2 years of follow-up (49). A more recent study reported that, after 6 months, 12% of 1569 patients with CLI needed amputation and 17.9% had persistent CLI (50).

Risk Factors for Worsening Peripheral Arterial Disease

Limited data are available concerning prognostic factors that play a role in the transition of asymptomatic PAD to symptomatic PAD. However, for the progression of symptomatic disease, smoking and diabetes have been shown to have an effect (9). Patients with IC who continued to smoke have been shown to develop CLI more often than patients with IC who quit smoking (51). Likewise, patients with IC who had a high load of lifetime smoking have required reconstructive vascular surgery 3 times more than those who smoked less (52). Finally, patients with IC who continued to smoke had higher amputation rates than those who quit (53).

Overall, patients with diabetes have more aggressive progression of PAD. Patients with IC and diabetes have been shown to have a 35% risk of sudden ischemia and 21% risk of major amputation compared with claudicants without diabetes who had a 19% risk of sudden ischemia and a 3% risk of major amputation (52,54). In addition, amputation or gangrene was 10 times more frequent in PAD subjects with diabetes than in those without diabetes (55).

The ABI has also been shown to be predictive of progressive PAD. In a prospective study of 1969 claudicants, an ABI <0.5 was the most significant predictor of deterioration of PAD assessed by arterial surgery or intervention (43). A low ABI has been associated with 2.4-fold higher risk of local atherosclerotic progression after 6.5 years of follow-up (56). There is also some evidence that the nature and symptoms of claudication might be related to disease progression. In Bloor's classic follow-up study, a patient with sudden onset of claudication was twice as likely to improve as a patient with gradual onset (57). Also, there is some evidence that claudication has a less severe course in women. Studies have reported that although the ratio between males and females is 2:1, in claudicants it increases to between 3:1 and 13:1 in later stages of the disease (58).

Peripheral Arterial Disease and Other Cardiovascular Diseases

Peripheral Arterial Disease and Co-Existing Cardiovascular Disease

The prognosis of patients with lower-extremity PAD is characterized by an increased risk of cardiovascular ischemic events, probably at least partly due to concomitant CAD and cerebrovascular disease in these patients. This has been confirmed by epidemiological research measuring the co-prevalence of PAD with other manifestations of atherosclerosis. The reported co-prevalence is highly dependent on the sensitivity of diagnostic tools used to define atherosclerotic disease, whether PAD, CHD, or stroke.

Overall, 40%-60% of claudicants suffer from co-existing CAD diagnosed by history of disease, clinical examination, or ECG, and 26%-50% of claudicants suffer from co-existing carotid disease diagnosed with duplex examination (9). Aronow and colleagues (59) studied the co-prevalence of PAD with other atherosclerotic manifestations in a long-term care facility. This study showed that of 468 patients with PAD, 58% had CAD and 34% had suffered from ischemic stroke (diagnosed with clinical history or ECG). Similar findings were reported in the UK Whitehall Study, which found the prevalence of cardiovascular disease in patients with IC to be 54% (4).

The Edinburgh Artery Study and the PARTNERS showed that when PAD was defined by ABI <0.9, 71% and 56% of subjects had co-existing cardiovascular disease, respectively (5,15). In the NHANES study, the prevalence of CHD was 24% and the prevalence of stroke 11.2% among those with ABI <0.9, whereas of those with normal ABI, 7.1% had CHD and 2.9% had stroke (14). In addition, the ABI was reported to correlate well with other measures of arterial disease in other vascular beds such as carotid intima media thickness and coronary artery calcium levels (60).

Intermittent Claudication

Patients with IC have been shown to have an increased risk of angina, heart failure, fatal and non-fatal myocardial infarction (MI), fatal and non-fatal stroke, cardiovascular death, and all-cause mortality, as reported by large-scale epidemiological studies (Table 1-2) (61). For example, the Helsinki study (3) found a 3-fold increase in the risk of cardiovascular mortality in male claudicants compared with males without claudication.

Asymptomatic Disease

People with asymptomatic atherosclerosis measured by the ABI or other noninvasive modalities also have an increased risk of cardiovascular morbidity and mortality. Table 1-3 summarizes results from prospective studies and shows that individuals with ABI <0.9 are at increased risk of experiencing either coronary or cerebrovascular events. Moreover, a recent

**Table 1-2.   All-Cause and Cardiovascular Mortality in Subjects with
Intermittent Claudication (IC) Assessed by the WHO Questionnaire**

Study	Population with IC (n)	Age (yrs)	Follow-Up (yrs)	Total Mortality (%)	CVD Mortality (%)
Helsinki Study (3)	122M	30-59	5	14.7	12.3
	93F			2.1	NR
Whitehall Study (4)	147M†	40-64	17	38.1	30.6
	175M‡			40.0	24.0
Quebec Vascular Study (7)	188 M	35–64	12	11.2	8.5
Edinburgh Artery Study (6,7)	73 MF	55-74	5	19.2	13.4

M: men, F: females, NR: not reported
†Probable IC ‡Possible IC

meta-analysis of nine studies that followed up subjects prospectively
showed that the sensitivity (the proportion of truly diseased persons who
are identified as diseased by the test under study) and specificity (the proportion of truly non-diseased persons who are so identified by the diagnostic test under study) of a low ABI (ABI <0.9) to predict CHD or stroke
were 16% and 92%, and for cardiovascular mortality were 41% and 88%, respectively (62). Finally, a low ABI has been shown to be a strong predictor of all-cause mortality (63).

In the Edinburgh Artery Study, after 5 years of follow-up, people with
an ABI <0.9 at baseline had an increased risk of non-fatal MI (relative risk
1.38), stroke (1.98), and cardiovascular death (1.85), after adjustment for
age, sex, coronary disease, and diabetes. A later report from this study, with
12 years follow-up, demonstrated that an ABI <0.9 had improved prediction of fatal MI over and above that of conventional risk factors (64). The
Framingham study of 251 men and 423 women aged 80 and older showed
that ABI <0.9 was associated with a 2-fold increase in the risk of stroke but
not with the risk of CHD (65). In addition, the US Cardiovascular Health
Study measured the ABI in adults older than 65 years of age and found that
an ABI <0.9 was significantly associated with both incident and recurrent
cardiovascular disease (66). Moreover, the ARIC study examined the relation between ABI and incident stroke after 7 years and reported a more
than 5-fold increase in the risk of stroke in people with ABI <0.8 (67).

The US Cardiovascular Health Study, along with the Strong Heart Study
in American Indians, recently examined the prognostic significance of high
ABI (68,69). As previously described, in subjects with diabetes the ABI is
artificially high due to arterial calcification. With that perception, high ABI
could be a measure of increased arterial stiffness and therefore predictive
of adverse cardiovascular results. Most epidemiologic studies have excluded subjects with increased ABI above 1.4 or 1.5 from their analyses.
The Cardiovascular Health Study and the Strong Heart Study did not make
these exclusions and have recently found a U-shaped relationship between

Table 1-3.   Prospective Studies of the Risk Ratio (95% CI) for People with ABI <0.9 for Development of Non-Fatal Coronary Heart Disease or Stroke in the General Population

Study	Population	Age (yrs)	Follow-Up (yrs)	Coronary Heart Disease	Stroke
				Risk Ratio of ABI <0.9 (95% CI)	
Edinburgh Artery Study (86)	1,592 MF	55-70	5	1.4 (0.9, 2.2)	2.0 (1.0, 3.8)†
Framingham offspring study (65)	251 M 423 F	80*	4	1.2 (0.7, 2.1)	2.0 (1.1, 3.7)‡
Honolulu Heart Program (26)	2,863 M	71-93	3-6	3.3 (2.2, 4.9) 2.7 (1.6, 4.5)	2.4 (1.5, 4.0)§ 2.0 (1.1, 3.5)
Cardiovascular Health Study (66)	5,888 MF	≥65	6	2.0 (1.4, 3.0)	1.6 (1.1, 2.3)
Atherosclerosis Risk in Communities Study (67)	14,839 MF	45-64	7	—	5.7 (2.8, 11.7) 1.9 (0.8, 4.8)‖
Belgian study (87)	2,023 M	40-55	10	5.0 (P = 0.006)	—

* mean age
† Adjusted for age, sex, coronary disease, and diabetes at baseline
‡ Adjusted for age, sex, and prevalent cardiovascular disease
§ PAD defined by ABI<0.8. First risk ratio adjusted for age and second for cardiovascular risk factors
‖ Age and sex adjusted

ABI and the risk of mortality; however, these results need replication from other studies (68,69).

Critical Limb Ischemia

In general, cardiovascular and all-cause mortality among those with CLI is high. In addition, patients with CLI have a 3-fold higher risk of future MI, stroke, and vascular death compared with patients with IC (70). There are few studies that have followed up subjects with CLI. In one study, 20% of patients with CLI died within a year (48). In another, 40%-70% died after 5 years of follow-up (71). Similar results were presented from a follow-up study in Italy: of 574 patients diagnosed with CLI, 21.9% died within 1 year (49). As expected, the overall incidence of vascular deaths was significantly higher than that of non-vascular deaths (34.5 vs. 8.5%).

Summary

PAD is a manifestation of atherosclerotic disease in the arteries to the legs. The clinical presentation of PAD spans a spectrum of individuals with asymptomatic disease, those who experience IC, and those with more severe symptoms of CLI.

Epidemiologic research has confirmed that PAD is a common condition that affects a large proportion of the adult population worldwide. The estimated prevalence of claudication ranges from 0.4% to 14.4%. The prevalence of asymptomatic disease diagnosed with noninvasive tests is much higher and ranges between 0.9% and 22%, with the ratio of symptomatic to asymptomatic ranging between 1:0.9 and 1:6. Risk factors for atherosclerosis such as age, cigarette smoking, diabetes, dyslipidemia, and hypertension increase the likelihood of developing lower-extremity PAD. Smoking and diabetes have also been associated with the progression of symptomatic disease.

The majority of patients with IC experience stabilization of their symptoms in 5 years and only 10%-15% ever develop CLI. The progression in the legs of those with asymptomatic disease is very little studied. However, both claudicants and those with asymptomatic disease are at increased risk of systemic cardiovascular events.

The diagnosis of PAD in epidemiologic studies is usually performed by noninvasive diagnostic tests. The ABI is the most commonly used noninvasive test and can be considered as an accurate and reliable marker of subclinical peripheral and generalized atherosclerosis in populations. Indeed, a decreased ABI (usually below 0.9) has been associated with increased risk of MI, stroke, and other manifestations of atherosclerosis and with other noninvasive tests of subclinical disease in other vascular beds.

Thus PAD is a common condition, especially if asymptomatic individuals are accounted for. However, the natural history of asymptomatic disease is not well established epidemiologically. Specific risk factors for the progression of asymptomatic disease need to be established to help the identification of seemingly healthy individuals who are at increased risk of experiencing a cardiovascular event and to provide insights into the early stages of disease development.

REFERENCES

1. Hirsch AT, Haskal ZJ, Hertzer NR, et al. Guidelines for the management of patients with peripheral arterial disease J Am Coll Cardiol. 2006;47:1239-312.
2. Dormandy J, Mahir M, Ascady G, et al. Fate of the patient with chronic leg ischaemia. A review article. J Cardiovasc Surg (Torino). 1989;30:50-7.
3. Reunanen A, Takkunen H, Aromaa A. Prevalence of intermittent claudication and its effect on mortality. Acta Med Scand. 1982;211:249-56.
4. Smith GD, Shipley MJ, Rose G. Intermittent claudication, heart disease risk factors, and mortality. The Whitehall Study. Circulation. 1990;82:1925-31.
5. Fowkes FG, Housley E, Cawood EH, et al. Edinburgh Artery Study: prevalence of asymptomatic and symptomatic peripheral arterial disease in the general population. Int J Epidemiol. 1991;20:384-92.
6. Kannel WB, Skinner JJ Jr., Schwartz MJ, Shurtleff D. Intermittent claudication. Incidence in the Framingham Study. Circulation. 1970;41:875-83.
7. Dagenais GR, Maurice S, Robitaille NM, et al. Intermittent claudication in Quebec men from 1974-1986: the Quebec Cardiovascular Study. Clin Invest Med. 1991;14:93-100.
8. Halperin JL. Evaluation of patients with peripheral vascular disease. Thromb Res. 2002; 106:V303-V311.

9. Dormandy JA, Rutherford RB. Management of peripheral arterial disease. TASC Working Group. TransAtlantic Inter-Society Concensus (TASC). J Vasc Surg. 2000;31:S1-S296.
10. Hiatt WR, Hoag S, Hammen RF. Effect of diagnistic criteria on the prevalence of peripheral arterial disease. Circulation. 1995;92:1472-9.
11. Stoffers HE, Rinkens PE, Kester AD, et al. The prevalence of asymptomatic and unrecognized peripheral arterial occlusive disease. Int J Epidemiol. 1996;25:282-90.
12. LeFevre FA, Corbacioglu C, Humphries AW, DeWolfe VG. Management of atherosclerosis obliterans of the extremities. JAMA. 1959;170:656-61.
13. Criqui MH, Fronek A, Barrett-Connor E, et al. The prevalence of peripheral arterial disease in a defined population. Circulation. 1985;71:510-5.
14. Selvin E, Erlinger TP. Prevalence of and risk factors for peripheral arterial disease in the United States: results from the National Health and Nutrition Examination Survey, 1999-2000. Circulation. 2004;110:738-43.
15. Hirsch AT, Criqui MH, Treat-Jacobson D, et al. Peripheral arterial disease detection, awareness, and treatment in primary care. JAMA. 2001;286:1317-24.
16. Hooi JD, Kester ADM, Stoffers HEJH, et al. Incidence of and risk factors for asymptomatic peripheral arterial occlusive disease: a longitudinal study. Am J Epidemiol. 2001;153:666-72.
17. The Vascular Surgery Society of Breat Britain and Ireland. Critical limb ischaemia: management and outcome. Report of a national survey. Eur J Vasc Endovasc Surg. 1995;10:108-13.
18. Catalano M. Epidemiology of critical limb isheamia: North Italian data. Eur J Med. 1993; 2:11-4.
19. Rothwell PM, Howard SC, Power DA, et al. Fibrinogen concentration and risk of ischemic stroke and acute coronary events in 5113 patients with transient ischemic attack and minor ischemic stroke. Stroke. 2004;35:2300-5.
20. Jensen SA, Vatten LJ, Myhre HO. The prevalence of chronic critical lower limb ischaemia in a population of 20,000 subjects 40-69 years of age. Eur J Vasc Endovasc Surg. 2006.
21. Freund KM, Belanger AJ, D'Agostino RB, Kannel WB. The health risks of smoking. The Framingham Study: 34 years of follow-up. Ann Epidemiol. 1993;3:417-24.
22. Fowkes FG, Housley E, Riemersma RA, et al. Smoking, lipids, glucose intolerance, and blood pressure as risk factors for peripheral atherosclerosis compared with ischemic heart disease in the Edinburgh Artery Study. Am J Epidemiol. 1992;135:331-40.
23. Willigendael EM, Teijink JAW, Bartelink ML, et al. Influence of smoking on incidence and prevalence of peripheral arterial disease. J Vasc Surg. 2004;40:1158-65.
24. Beks PJ, Mackaay AJ, de Neeling JN, et al. Peripheral arterial disease in relation to glycaemic level in an elderly Caucasian population: the Hoorn study. Diabetologia. 1995;38: 86-96.
25. Meijer WT, Hoes AW, Rutgers D, et al. Peripheral arterial disease in the elderly: The Rotterdam Study. Arterioscler Thromb Vasc Biol. 1998;18:185-92.
26. Abbott RD, Petrovitch H, Rodriguez BL, et al. Ankle/brachial blood pressure in men >70 years of age and the risk of coronary heart disease. Am J Cardiol. 2000;86:280-4.
27. Jude EB, Oyibo SO, Chalmers N, Boulton AJM. Peripheral arterial disease in diabetic and nondiabetic patients: a comparison of severity and outcome. Diabetes Care. 2001;24: 1433-7.
28. Luscher TF, Creager MA, Beckman JA, Cosentino F. Diabetes and vascular disease: pathophysiology, clinical consequences, and medical therapy: part II. Circulation. 2003;108: 1655-61.
29. Brand FN, Abbott RD, Kannel WB. Diabetes, intermittent claudication, and risk of cardiovascular events. The Framingham Study. Diabetes. 1989;38:504-9.
30. Criqui MH, Browner D, Fronek A, et al. Peripheral arterial disease in large vessels is epidemiologically distinct from small vessel disease. An analysis of risk factors. Am J Epidemiol. 1989;129:1110-9.
31. Ridker PM, Stampfer MJ, Rifai N. Novel risk factors for systemic atherosclerosis: a comparison of C-reactive protein, fibrinogen, homocysteine, lipoprotein(a), and standard cholesterol screening as predictors of peripheral arterial disease. JAMA. 2001;285:2481-5.
32. Duffield RG, Lewis B, Miller NE, et al. Treatment of hyperlipidaemia retards progression of symptomatic femoral atherosclerosis. A randomised controlled trial. Lancet. 1983;2:639-42.
33. Makin A, Lip GY, Silverman S, Beevers DG. Peripheral vascular disease and hypertension: a forgotten association? J Hum Hypertens. 2001;15:447-54.

34. Newman AB, Siscovick DS, Manolio TA, et al. Ankle-arm index as a marker of atherosclerosis in the Cardiovascular Health Study. Cardiovascular Heart Study (CHS) Collaborative Research Group. Circulation. 1993;88:837-45.

35. Kennedy M, Solomon C, Manolio TA, et al. Risk factors for declining ankle-brachial index in men and women 65 years or older: the Cardiovascular Health Study. Arch Intern Med. 2005;165:1896-902.

36. Smith FB, Lee AJ, Hau CM, et al. Plasma fibrinogen, haemostatic factors and prediction of peripheral arterial disease in the Edinburgh Artery Study. Blood Coagul Fibrinolysis. 2000;11:43-50.

37. Pradhan AD, Rifai N, Ridker PM. Soluble intercellular adhesion molecule-1, soluble vascular adhesion molecule-1, and the development of symptomatic peripheral arterial disease in men. Circulation. 2002;106:820-5.

38. Tzoulaki I, Murray GD, Lee AJ, et al. C-reactive protein, interleukin-6, and soluble adhesion molecules as predictors of progressive peripheral atherosclerosis in the general population: Edinburgh Artery Study. Circulation. 2005;112:976-83.

39. Planas A, Clara A, Pou JM, et al. Relationship of obesity distribution and peripheral arterial occlusive disease in elderly men. Int J Obes Relat Metab Disord. 2001;25:1068-70.

40. Housley E, Leng GC, Donnan PT, Fowkes FGR. Physical-Activity and Risk of Peripheral Arterial-Disease in the General-Population - Edinburgh-Artery-Study. J Epidemiol Community Health. 1993;47:475-80.

41. Criqui MH, Vargas V, Denenberg JO, et al. Ethnicity and peripheral arterial disease: the San Diego population study. Circulation. 2005;112:2703-7.

42. Zheng ZJ, Rosamond WD, Chambless LE, et al. Lower extremity arterial disease assessed by ankle-brachial index in a middle-aged population of African Americans and whites: the Atherosclerosis Risk in Communities (ARIC) Study. Am J Prev Med. 2005;29:42-9.

43. Dormandy JA, Murray GD. The fate of the claudicant: a prospective study of 1969 claudicants. Eur J Vasc Surg. 1991;5:131-3.

44. Peabody CN, Kannel WB, McNamara PM. Intermittent claudication. Surgical significance. Arch Surg. 1974;109:693-7.

45. Imparato AM, Kim GE, Davidson T, Crowley JG. Intermittent claudication: its natural course. Surgery. 1975;78:795-9.

46. Widmer LK, Da Silva A. Historical perspectives and the Basle study. In: Fowkes FGR, ed. Epidemiology of Peripheral Vascular Disease. London: Springer-Verlag; 1991. p. 69-83.

47. Smith FB, Lee AJ, Price JF, et al. Changes in ankle brachial index in symptomatic and asymptomatic subjects in the general population. J Vasc Surg. 2003;38:1323-30.

48. Wolfe JN. Defining the outcome of critical ischaemia: a one year prospective study. Br J Surg. 1986;73:321.

49. The ICAI group. Long-term mortality and its predictors in patients with critical leg ischaemia. The I.C.A.I. Group (Gruppo di Studio dell'Ischemia Cronica Critica degli Arti Inferiori). The Study Group of Criticial Chronic Ischemia of the Lower Exremities. Eur J Vasc Endovasc Surg. 1997;14:91-5.

50. Bertele V, Roncaglioni MC, Pangrazzi J, et al. Clinical outcome and its predictors in 1560 patients with critical leg ischaemia. Chronic Critical Leg Ischaemia Group. Eur J Vasc Endovasc Surg. 1999;18:401-10.

51. Jonason T, Bergstrom R. Cessation of smoking in patients with intermittent claudication. Effects on the risk of peripheral vascular complications, myocardial infarction and mortality. Acta Med Scand. 1987;221:253-60.

52. Cronenwett JL, Warner KG, Zelenock GB, et al. Intermittent claudication. Current results of nonoperative management. Arch Surg. 1984;119:430-6.

53. Lassila R, Lepantalo M. Cigarette smoking and the outcome after lower limb arterial surgery. Acta Chir Scand. 1988;154:635-40.

54. McDaniel MD, Cronenwett JL. Basic data related to the natural history of intermittent claudication. Ann Vasc Surg. 1989;3:273-7.

55. Dormandy J, Heeck L, Vig S. Predicting which patients will develop chronic critical leg ischemia. Semin Vasc Surg. 1999;12:138-41.

56. Jelnes R, Gaardsting O, Hougaard JK, et al. Fate in intermittent claudication: outcome and risk factors. Br Med J (Clin Res Ed). 1986;293:1137-40.

57. Bloor K. Natural history of arteriosclerosi of the lower extremities. Ann Roy Coll Surg Eng. 1961;28:36-51.
58. Fowkes FG. Epidemiology of peripheral arterial disease. In: Lowe GDO, editor. Texbook of vascular medicine. 1991. p. 149-58.
59. Aronow WS, Ahn C. Prevalence of coexistence of coronary artery disease, peripheral arterial disease, and atherothrombotic brain infarction in men and women > or = 62 years of age. Am J Cardiol. 1994;74:64-5.
60. McDermott MM, Liu K, Criqui MH, et al. Ankle-brachial index and subclinical cardiac and carotid disease: The multi-ethnic study of atherosclerosis. Am J Epidemiol. 2005;162:33-41.
61. Ouriel K. Peripheral arterial disease. Lancet. 2001;358:1257-64.
62. Doobay AV, Anand SS. Sensitivity and specificity of the ankle-brachial index to predict future cardiovascular outcomes: a systematic review. Arterioscler Thromb Vasc Biol. 2005; 25:1463-9.
63. Heald CL, Fowkes FGR, Murray GD, Price JF. Risk of mortality and cardiovascular disease associated with the ankle-brachial index: Systematic review. Atherosclerosis.In Press, Corrected Proof.
64. Lee AJ, Price JF, Russell MJ, et al. Improved prediction of fatal myocardial infarction using the ankle brachial index in addition to conventional risk factors: the Edinburgh Artery Study. Circulation. 2004;110:3075-80.
65. Murabito JM, Evans JC, Larson MG, et al. The ankle-brachial index in the elderly and risk of stroke, coronary disease, and death: the Framingham Study. Arch Intern Med. 2003; 163:1939-42.
66. Newman AB, Shemanski L, Manolio TA, et al. Ankle-arm index as a predictor of cardiovascular disease and mortality in the Cardiovascular Health Study. The Cardiovascular Health Study Group. Arterioscler Thromb Vasc Biol. 1999;19:538-45.
67. Tsai AW, Folsom AR, Rosamond WD, Jones DW. Ankle-brachial index and 7-year ischemic stroke incidence: the ARIC study. Stroke. 2001;32:1721-4.
68. O'Hare AM, Katz R, Shlipak MG, et al. Mortality and cardiovascular risk across the ankle-arm index spectrum: results from the Cardiovascular Health Study. Circulation. 2006;113: 388-93.
69. Resnick HE, Lindsay RS, McDermott MM, et al. Relationship of high and low ankle brachial index to all-cause and cardiovascular disease mortality: the Strong Heart Study. Circulation. 2004;109:733-9.
70. Novo S, Coppola G, Milio G. Critical limb ischemia: definition and natural history. Curr Drug Targets Cardiovasc Haematol Disord. 2004;4:219-25.
71. Dormandy J, Heeck L, Vig S. The fate of patients with critical leg ischemia. Semin Vasc Surg. 1999;12:142-7.
72. Bothig S, Metelitsa VI, Barth W, et al. Prevalence of ischaemic heart disease, arterial hypertension and intermittent claudication, and distribution of risk factors among middle-aged men in Moscow and Berlin. Cor Vasa. 1976;18:104-18.
73. Hughson WG, Mann JI, Garrod A. Intermittent claudication: prevalence and risk factors. BMJ. 1978;1:1379-81.
74. Schroll M, Munck O. Estimation of peripheral arteriosclerotic disease by ankle blood pressure measurements in a population study of 60-year-old men and women. J Chronic Dis. 1981;34:261-9.
75. Gofin R, Kark JD, Friedlander Y, et al. Peripheral vascular disease in a middle-aged population sample. The Jerusalem Lipid Research Clinic Prevalence Study. Isr J Med Sci. 1987;23:157-67.
76. Dewhurst G, Wood DA, Walker F, et al. A population survey of cardiovascular disease in elderly people: design, methods and prevalence results. Age Ageing. 1991;20:353-60.
77. Mittelmark M, Psaty BM, Rautaharju PM, et al. Prevalence of cardiovascular diseases among older adults. The Cardiovascular Health Study. Am J Epidemiol. 1993;137:311-7.
78. Bowlin SJ, Medalie JH, Flocke SA, et al. Intermittent claudication in 8343 men and 21-year specific mortality follow-up. Ann Epidemiol. 1997;7:180-7.
79. Bainton D, Sweetnam P, Baker I, et al. Peripheral Vascular-Disease - Consequence for Survival and Association with Risk-Factors in the Speedwell Prospective Heart-Disease Study. Br Heart J. 1994;72:128-32.

80. **Wilt TJ, Davis BR, Meyers DG, et al.** Prevalence and correlates of symptomatic peripheral atherosclerosis in individuals with coronary heart disease and cholesterol levels less than 240 mg/dL: baseline results from the Cholesterol and Recurrent Events (CARE) Study. Angiology. 1996;47:533-41.

81. **Ness J, Aronow WS, Ahn C.** Risk factors for symptomatic peripheral arterial disease in older persons in an academic hospital-based geriatrics practice. J Am Geriatr Soc. 2000;48:312-4.

82. **Murabito JM, Evans JC, Nieto K, et al.** Prevalence and clinical correlates of peripheral arterial disease in the Framingham Offspring Study. Am Heart J. 2002;143:961-5.

83. **Brevetti G, Oliva G, Silvestro A, et al.** Prevalence, risk factors and cardiovascular comorbidity of symptomatic peripheral arterial disease in Italy. Atherosclerosis. 2004;175:131-8.

84. **Diehm C, Schuster A, Allenberg JR, et al.** High prevalence of peripheral arterial disease and co-morbidity in 6880 primary care patients: cross-sectional study. Atherosclerosis. 2004; 172:95-105.

85. **Zheng ZJ, Sharrett AR, Chambless LE, et al.** Associations of ankle-brachial index with clinical coronary heart disease, stroke and preclinical carotid and popliteal atherosclerosis: the Atherosclerosis Risk in Communities (ARIC) Study. Atherosclerosis. 1997;131:115-25.

86. **Leng GC, Lee AJ, Fowkes FG, et al.** Incidence, natural history and cardiovascular events in symptomatic and asymptomatic peripheral arterial disease in the general population. Int J Epidemiol. 1996;25:1172-81.

87. **Kornitzer M, Dramaix M, Sobolski J, et al.** Ankle/arm pressure index in asymptomatic middle-aged males: an independent predictor of ten-year coronary heart disease mortality. Angiology. 1995;46:211-9.

KEY REFERENCES

Ouriel K. Peripheral arterial disease. Lancet. 2001;358:1257-64. *A narrative review on epidemiology, risk factors and management of PAD.*

Dormandy JA, Rutherford RB. Management of peripheral arterial disease (PAD). TASC Working Group. TransAtlantic Inter-Society Consensus (TASC). J Vasc Surg. 2000;31:S1-S296. *An excellent review on PAD.*

Leng GC, Lee AJ, Fowkes FG, et al. Incidence, natural history and cardiovascular events in symptomatic and asymptomatic peripheral arterial disease in the general population. Int J Epidemiol. 1996;25:1172-81. *The incidence and natural history of PAD as evaluated in the 5 years follow-up of the Edinburgh Artery Study.*

Hirsch AT, Criqui MH, Treat-Jacobson D, et al. Peripheral arterial disease detection, awareness, and treatment in primary care. JAMA. 2001;286:1317-24. *A multicenter, cross-sectional study conducted at 27 sites in 25 cities and 350 primary care practices throughout the United States. The frequency of PAD detection, physician and patient awareness of PAD diagnosis, treatment intensity in PAD patients compared with treatment of other forms of cardiovascular disease and with patients without clinical evidence of atherosclerosis were evaluated.*

Doobay AV, Anand SS. Sensitivity and specificity of the ankle-brachial index to predict future cardiovascular outcomes: a systematic review. Arterioscler Thromb Vasc Biol. 2005;25:1463-9. *The objective of this review was to determine the sensitivity and specificity of an ankle-brachial index <0.90 to predict future cardiovascular events, including coronary heart disease, stroke, and death.*

Meijer WT, Hoes AW, Rutgers D, et al. Peripheral arterial disease in the elderly: The Rotterdam Study. Arterioscler Thromb Vasc Biol. 1998;18:185-92. *Results from the Rotterdam study showing that prevalence of an ABI <0.9 in the elderly is high whereas the prevalence of IC is rather low, although both prevalences clearly increased with advancing age.*

Selvin E, Erlinger TP. Prevalence of and risk factors for peripheral arterial disease in the United States: results from the National Health and Nutrition Examination Survey, 1999-2000. Circulation. 2004;110:738-43. *This study provided nationally representative prevalence estimates of PAD in the United States, revealing that PAD affects more than 5 million adults.*

Chapter 2

Differential Diagnosis and Office Evaluation of Peripheral Arterial Disease

THOM W. ROOKE, MD

1. What are historical clues to PAD?
2. What are the physical examination findings?
3. Which office-based diagnostic tests confirm PAD?
4. What diseases mimic PAD?
5. When is it necessary to refer for further testing?

Peripheral arterial disease (PAD) (atherosclerosis involving the lower extremities) is important for two major reasons: 1) It may produce symptoms (ranging from minor claudication to ulceration, gangrene, and potential limb loss), bringing the patient to his or her health care provider for further evaluation; and 2) PAD is a marker for atherosclerosis in other arterial distributions, such as the coronaries or carotids.

Because PAD is such a common condition with major implications, it is essential that health care providers search for it in appropriate settings and familiarize themselves with the basic physical examination and the simple objective tests available for detecting this disease.

Historical Clues to Peripheral Arterial Disease

Few pathological entities can be diagnosed by history alone more reliably than PAD (1). For example, many patients with PAD present with claudication. Derived from a Latin term meaning "to limp," vasculogenic claudication is readily identified as a symptom of PAD. With typical claudication, the patient is entirely asymptomatic at rest or with standing. Pain is produced by walking or using the lower extremities. This pain typically affects a specific part of the leg or legs (although the entire lower extremity may be affected); it comes on with a predictable walking distance or amount of work; and it is readily relieved by a short period of rest. The patient does not need to sit or lie down while resting to experience relief. Although ambient factors may affect these symptoms (i.e., they may come on earlier in cold weather, when walking up hill, etc.), it is the consistency of this sequence that typifies true claudication. Unfortunately, patients do not necessarily volunteer their symptoms of claudication (or other sequelae of PAD), so the provider may need to prod them during the history. One approach is to focus on five specific questions that help to elucidate the presence of PAD.

1. Does the patient have risk factors for arteriosclerosis obliterans (ASO)?

Common risk factors should be assessed in every patient. In patients of an appropriate age (typically over 40), health care providers should always inquire about family history (for PAD or other atherosclerotic diseases), smoking history, and the presence of diabetes or hypertension. If diabetes or hypertension is present, additional questions should be asked about the type of treatment the patient is receiving and the effectiveness of therapy.

2. Are there known PAD/blockages in the leg or blood vessel problems, etc.?

Not surprisingly, patients can often tell you whether they have PAD, and this should therefore be one of the first questions asked; a "yes" to this question allows the provider to quickly focus on other areas of interest. The patient can generally tell you whether they have been told by other physicians that they have blockages in their leg arteries, or whether they have had bypass operations, angioplasty, stenting, etc. Medically astute patients may be able to give you considerable detail about their diagnosis and previous treatments, including type and location of grafts, presence of stents, previous medical therapies, etc.

3. Is there atherosclerosis in other vascular beds?

When attempting to determine whether specific lower-extremity symptoms may be due to PAD, it is extremely useful to ascertain whether the patient has known atherosclerosis in other distributions such as the coronary or carotids. If so, it raises the odds of PAD as a cause of the patient's complaints.

4. Are there signs or symptoms of PAD?

PAD, in its mild forms, may be entirely asymptomatic. As noted above, when it becomes symptomatic, claudication is the predominant symptom. Health care providers need to take a detailed history of this manifestation whenever it is suspected. Questions to be asked should include:

- Where do the symptoms occur (buttocks, thighs, calves, elsewhere)? The location of symptoms is often a reliable predictor of the location of arterial blockage.
- What does the pain feel like? (Is it an achy, crampy sensation? A shooting pain? Diffuse burning?). The nature of the pain can be helpful. For example, pains that shoot down the leg are typically associated with nerve problems such as sciatica and much less commonly with vascular problems. Similarly, pains that develop or disappear within a few seconds are unlikely to be vascular.
- How far can the patient walk? (As noted earlier, claudication is quite predictable and generally consistent. Patients can usually describe a typical activity or distance that precipitates their symptoms).
- What factors relieve the claudication? (Claudication should be relieved with 2 to 3 minutes of rest. Importantly, the patient can generally stand and recover. If the patient describes a need to sit down, change positions, etc., it raises the possibility of other diagnoses such as pseudoclaudication from spinal stenosis).

In addition to claudication, other signs and symptoms of PAD that should be inquired about include the following:

- **Sensation:** Limbs with PAD should be assessed for sensory neuropathy, particularly if diabetes is present. If sensation is reduced, the risk of skin damage increases markedly;
- **Other Pains**: In addition to symptoms that mimic claudication, there may be other types of discomfort that affect the leg and can be associated with PAD (2) or confused with pain caused by PAD. As discussed later, spinal stenosis and trochanteric bursitis may produce hip pains that can be confused with claudication;
- **Appearance**: Patients must be asked about color, presence of edema, changes in hair growth, skin breakdown, and any other aspect of the appearance of their limb that may be related to PAD;
- **Ulcer/skin breakdown**: This should be specifically inquired about. If the patient has a history of previous ulceration or skin breakdown, additional questioning should focus on the nature of the precipitating event (if any), the measures used to heal the wound, the length of time required for wound healing, and any measures taken to prevent future recurrences, etc.

5. Do your symptoms limit your lifestyle?

This is perhaps the most important question to ask with regard to claudication. In some patients (i.e., the proverbial couch potato), the amount of claudication that can be tolerated without significantly impacting the patient's lifestyle is often amazing. Some patients are content as long as their fingers can continue to work the TV remote. In these patients, it does not always make sense to pursue aggressive measures (such as revascularization) to improve their minimal symptoms, even when the disease is objectively quite severe. As long as the limbs are not in ischemic jeopardy, it may be best to pursue less aggressive measures. In contrast, extremely active patients may find that relatively mild PAD produces symptoms that adversely affect their lifestyle enough to warrant intervention (for example, patients who enjoy running, golfing, hiking, etc., may not be able to pursue these activities if mild PAD produces symptoms).

Physical Examination Findings

While subtleties in the vascular examination may be best appreciated by those who specialize in vascular diseases, all health care providers should be able to perform a basic vascular examination. Multiple senses, including touch, hearing, and vision are used in the examination process (3).

Palpation

The most important aspect of palpation is to evaluate the peripheral pulses (Figure 2-1). These should be examined not just in the legs (anterior and posterior tibial, popliteal, and femoral), but also in the upper extremity (brachial, radial, and ulnar), neck (carotid), and abdomen (palpation for aortic aneurysm). When appropriate, inspection of the upper extremity should include Allen testing (i.e., checking for hand perfusion while manually occluding the radial artery at the wrist) to determine ulnar patency (Figure 2-2). Depending on the depth and strength of the particular pulse in question, the examiner may need to use certain "tricks" to optimally appreciate pulsations; these include varying the intensity of fingertip pressure, using multiple fingers, altering the patient's position, etc. With practice, all of the aforementioned pulses should be identifiable on a routine basis.

Vascular specialists have devised elaborate schemes for grading pulses (4), based on scales of 0 to 4+ (normal) or 5+ (aneurysm), but for most health care practitioners it is adequate to identify whether a pulse is present, absent, or aneurysmal. The use of adjectives is helpful in describing the important characteristics of the pulse (booming, barely palpable, weak, etc.). Although the interpretation of these adjectives may vary from examiner to examiner, the variability is probably no more than it is for many

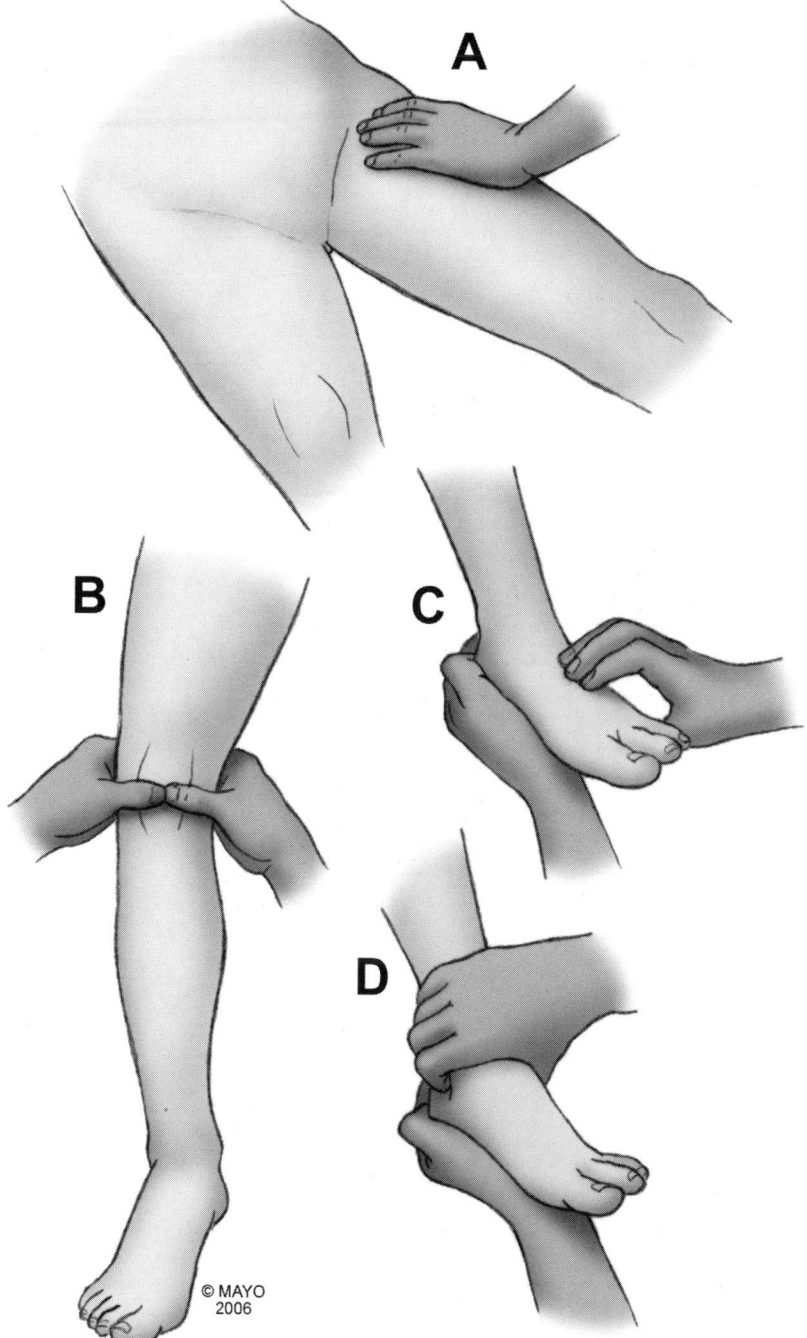

Figure 2-1.   Technique for palpating the A) femoral, B) popliteal, C) dorsalis pedis, and D) posterior tibial pulses.

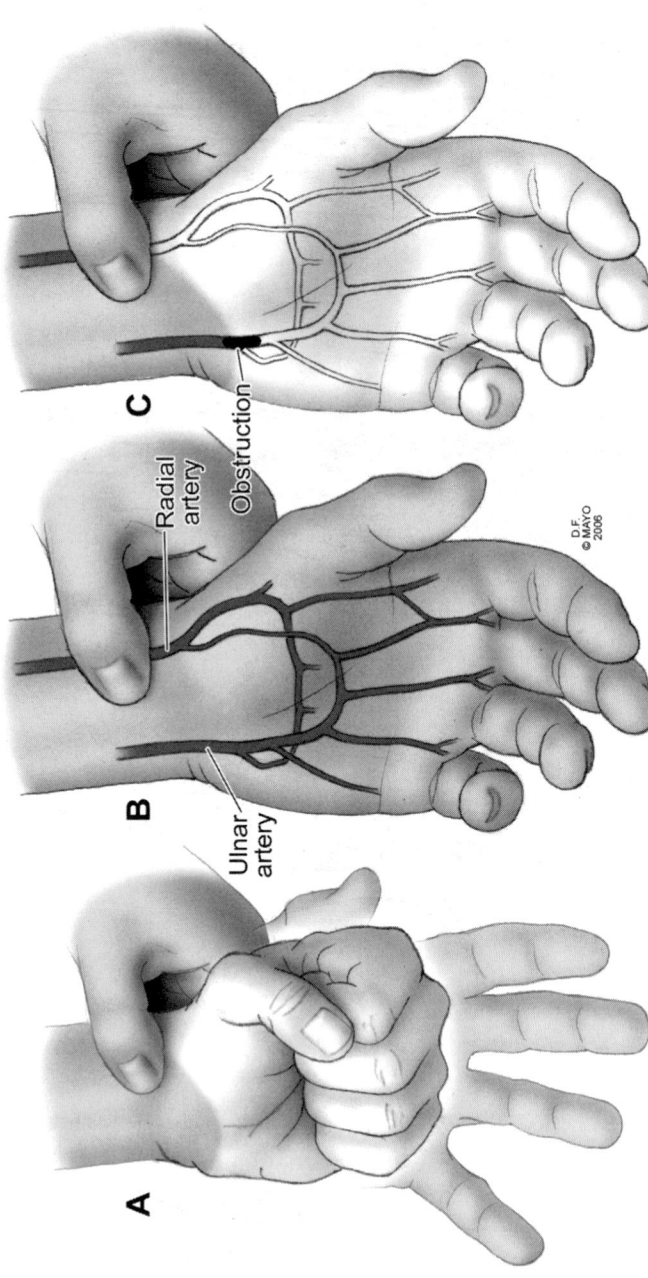

Figure 2-2. Technique for performing the Allen test. A) The fist is squeezed multiple times while the radial artery is manually compressed. B) The hand is relaxed while radial artery compression is maintained. If the ulnar artery is patent, refilling occurs promptly. C) If the ulnar artery or palmar branch vessels are occluded, refilling is absent or delayed.

other characteristics that are described using common medical adjectives. Most importantly, by using adjectives, the examiner sets the stage for being able to perform meaningful serial studies over time (i.e., the examiner knows what she meant by a "booming" pulse, and if she does not notice this in the future, it suggests that the examination may have changed).

Other qualities that can be assessed using palpation include skin temperature and texture. A note of caution with temperature: coolness of the skin does not necessarily imply PAD. Many "normal" limbs are cool to the touch because of transient vasoconstriction or other physiological phenomenon. Women, in particular, often have cool limbs owing to reduced cutaneous blood flow (this occurs on a physiological basis) (5). Skin texture, including characteristics such as thickness, thinness, roughness, presence or absence of edema (pitting), and other characteristics should be described when appropriate.

Auscultation

Using a stethoscope, areas of interest can be evaluated for bruits. A bruit is produced by turbulent blood flow and may be associated with stenotic lesions, aneurysms, or other anatomic abnormalities (a palpable bruit is called a "thrill"). Although bruits are most commonly heard over diseased carotid arteries, it is possible to hear them in the abdomen (reflecting mesenteric, renal, or aortic turbulence), and in the inguinal areas (iliac turbulence). Even when anatomical lesions are present in other places, bruits may be more difficult to appreciate. The value of hearing a bruit is that it may indicate the presence of disease sufficient to create turbulence but not so severe that it attenuates the pulse. It can also confirm the presence of PAD when one is uncertain whether the pulse is reduced.

Inspection

As Yogi Berra put it, "You can observe a lot by watching." What is true for baseball is true for vascular disease. Visual inspection is a key component of the physical examination of PAD. For example, color changes may provide a clue as to the presence or severity of PAD. In some cases, provocative maneuvers may enhance the underlying color changes. Pallor is a sign of impaired arterial inflow, and this can be enhanced by elevating the limb, typically for 30 to 60 seconds. Cyanosis and rubor reflect venous congestion (often seen in the presence of arterial inflow) and are enhanced by placing the limbs in a dependent position. Elevation pallor and dependent rubor are therefore two signs of significant occlusive disease (Figure 2-3). Other color changes, including livedo reticularis (a lacy, spiderweb-type pattern that appears over the legs in association with certain vascular conditions such as vasculitis, atheroemboli, and others) may be evident and can often be accentuated by having the patient stand. Other findings commonly noted on

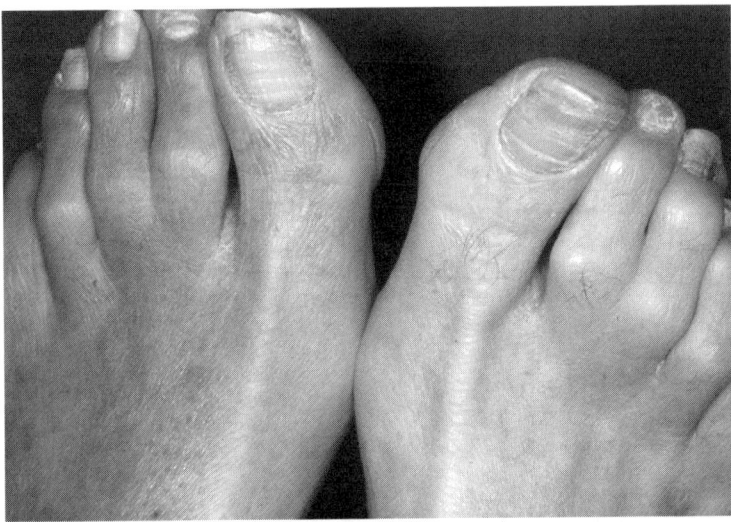

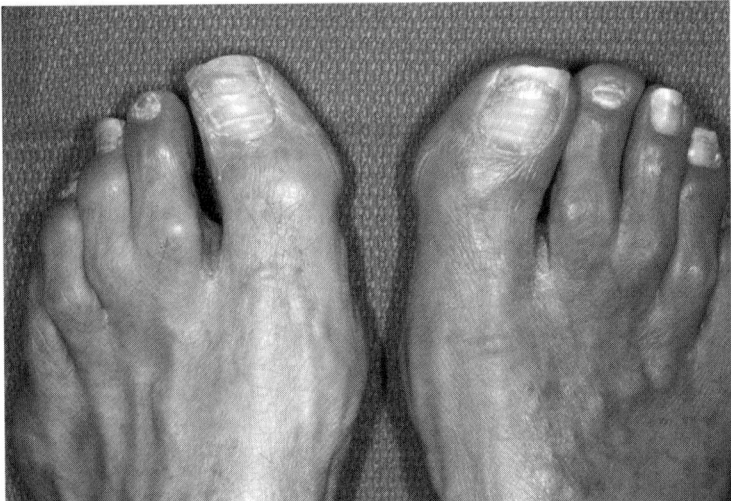

Figure 2-3. Elevation pallor/dependence rubor. With the patient in a supine position, the legs are elevated to 45 degrees. If arterial insufficiency is present, the feet will become pale (A) over the next 60 seconds (elevation pallor). Following this, the patient is asked to sit up and hang their feet in a dependent position. The subsequent appearance of rubor (B) is another indication of arterial compromise.

inspection include ulcerations, petechiae, infarcted areas, and various trophic skin changes. Trophic changes include thinning or thickening of the skin in response to chronically inadequate blood flow, changes in hair growth, callus formation, etc. Whenever significant PAD is suspected, it is important to inspect the feet carefully, including the area between the toes, where occult skin breakdown or "kissing ulcers" may develop (Figure 2-4).

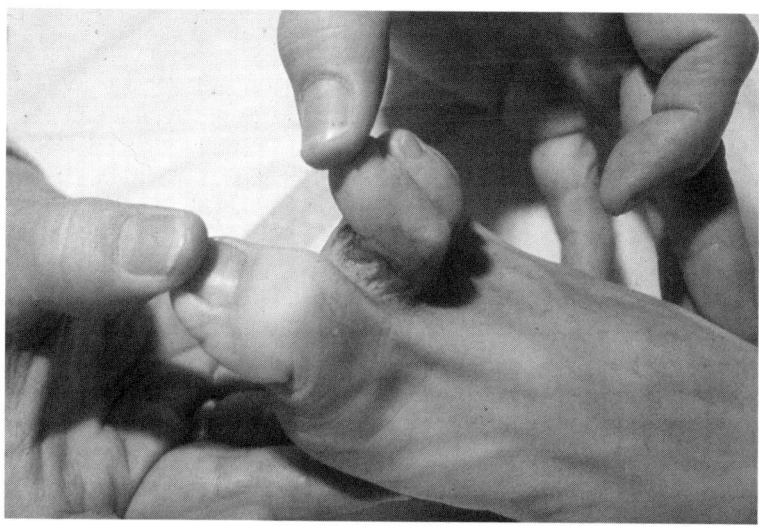

Figure 2-4. Foot inspection. The areas between toes should be examined for occult ulcers.

Office-Based Evaluation of Peripheral Arterial Disease

The most important "test" for assessing PAD is the physical examination, but in many settings it is necessary to perform more objective testing. At the far extreme, this can involve imaging (angiography, computerized tomography [CT] angiography, magnetic resonance [MR] angiography), which may be invasive and will always be expensive (see Chapter 4). Another approach is to evaluate the patient in a conventional noninvasive "vascular laboratory" (see Chapter 3). These laboratories, typically based on duplex ultrasonography but often with additional hemodynamic or functional tests available, are the mainstay of formal objective vascular testing.

Within the office setting, it is possible to make important, objective measurements using simple tools. The most essential of these is the hand-held continuous wave (CW) Doppler, a device that has been available to the clinician for decades. Simple Dopplers, most of which cost less than $500, provide an audio output of the arterial Doppler signal. A CW Doppler can be used for detecting pulses when they are not palpable (because of edema, arterial obstructions, etc.), and the shape of the waveform can be assessed. In its simplest form, a normal arterial Doppler signal should be triphasic or biphasic; when interrogation occurs distal to a hemodynamically significant lesion, the signal is typically monophasic (see Chapter 3). By interrogating a limb at multiple sites, it is possible to identify the presence and location of hemodynamically significant lesions.

Although the handheld CW Doppler has utility for finding obscure pulses and assessing the presence of arterial disease (by looking for waveform abnormalities), it is most useful in the office setting when combined with a blood pressure cuff. By measuring the systolic arm pressures and the ankle pressures using a cuff and a Doppler, one can obtain the ankle-brachial pressure index (ABI). This assessment, explained in detail in Chapter 3, allows the primary care physician to make an office-based measurement that is accurate, reproducible, sensitive, and specific for the diagnosis of arterial disease. The test is performed by obtaining the ankle blood pressures (usually the higher of the anterior or posterior tibial blood pressures) and dividing this by the higher of the two arm (brachial) systolic pressures. The resulting index is normally greater than one, and it decreases as PAD worsens. In situations where the resting study is normal but the history is highly suggestive of PAD, the patient can be exercised (using a walk in the hallway or tiptoe maneuvers) to help increase the sensitivity of the examination (the pressure measurements need to be repeated immediately at the completion of exercise).

Office-based studies of the lower-extremity arteries may yield valuable information. If a study is negative, it reinforces a clinical impression that PAD is neither present nor responsible for the patient's complaints. If it is positive, it may confirm PAD but can also give important information about the severity of the disease. As noted earlier, the presence of PAD predicts the occurrence of atherosclerosis in other arterial distributions, and as the severity of PAD increases, the overall mortality risk for the patient also increases (6). Surprisingly, a simple office-based test may predict overall cardiovascular mortality better than many other tests that are more elaborate, expensive, or invasive.

The issue of arterial screening is controversial when applied to formal (and increasingly for-profit) screening programs or vascular laboratories, but there is no controversy in the office setting. All patients of appropriate age should be screened for arterial disease via the history and physical examination. In patients where risk factors (i.e., diabetes, smoking, family history, hypertension, etc.) or physical findings (absent pulses, etc.) raise the possibility of occult PAD, objective testing (such as handheld Doppler interrogation or ABI measurement) in the primary care setting is absolutely appropriate. The fact that the patient is not complaining of symptoms consistent with PAD should not dissuade the health care provider from performing a screening examination in a clinically appropriate setting.

Diseases That Mimic Peripheral Arterial Disease

A boring laundry list of conditions that mimic PAD can be made more tolerable by dividing them into two categories: 1) non-atherosclerotic arterial diseases, and 2) non-arterial diseases.

Non-Atherosclerotic Arterial Diseases

These important but fortunately uncommon entities are often mistakenly assumed to be PAD when they first present. They can be subcategorized according to the fundamental abnormality. For example:

1. Structural abnormalities: these include entities such as fibromuscular dysplasia, connective tissue disorders (Ehlers-Danlos, pseudoxanthoma elasticum, etc.), congenital abnormalities (including coarctation of the aorta and atresia of various arteries), and many others. These conditions, many of which are congenital, frequently present at an earlier age than PAD, but in some patients they may not become manifest until the patient is over 40.

2. Inflammatory conditions: Many types of vasculitis may be mistaken for PAD, but the most common mimics are giant cell arteritis (temporal arteritis) and Takayasu's arteritis. Because of its propensity to affect older individuals, giant cell arteritis in particular may be confused with PAD. In younger patients, involvement of the distal aorta and iliac arteritis by Takayasu's disease is relatively common and may mimic premature atherosclerosis.

3. Thromboembolic disease: Clot formation within a lower-extremity blood vessel (thrombosis) or, more commonly, an embolus from the heart may produce arterial obstruction that can, in some circumstances, mimic PAD. In general, the manifestations of thromboembolic disease are more acute than PAD, but when subclinical or serial thromboembolic events occur, the result may be the slow accumulation of blockages that eventually become clinically evident and are easily mistaken for PAD.

4. Impingement/entrapment: In the lower extremity, this is most commonly seen in the popliteal region, where a variety of anatomical variations can lead to an entity known as "popliteal entrapment." In this condition, foot flexion (either plantar or dorsiflexion) may tense muscles in the leg and compress the popliteal artery, causing intermittent ischemia during running or walking. Because this symptom is indeed a form of claudication, it is often assumed to be due to PAD. However, patients with impingement or entrapment syndromes are typically younger and healthier than the usual population with PAD.

5. Others: A variety of obscure diseases can mimic PAD. An encyclopedic recounting of these is unnecessary for the general practitioner, but they include conditions such as popliteal cystic disease (in which mucinous cysts form in the wall of the popliteal and other arteries, compressing the lumen and producing obstruction); iliac endofibrosis, seen in competitive bicyclists; sclerosis of the aorta and iliac vessels caused by pelvic radiation (for neoplastic disease); and numerous others.

Non-Arterial Disease

In addition to diseases that mimic PAD by causing arterial blockage or disruption, there are other diseases that mimic PAD even though they have no effect on the arteries. A classic but rare entity is venous claudication, which occasionally occurs when the veins leading out of the leg become obstructed to the point where venous hypertension limits arterial inflow. As a result, the patient may "claudicate" during activities involving the leg. A much more common mimic of PAD is "pseudoclaudication," which is caused by spinal stenosis. In this condition, compression of the spinal cord causes symptoms during ambulation that may be indistinguishable from those produced by PAD. These two diseases can often be differentiated from each other during the post-exercise phase. With claudication, patients achieve relief simply by standing and resting. In contrast, patients with pseudoclaudication often need to assume a different posture for relief; this may entail leaning forward (which can relieve pressure on the lumbar region), sitting, or laying down, etc. In extreme cases, prolonged standing alone may trigger leg symptoms with pseudoclaudication; this virtually never occurs with vasculogenic claudication caused by PAD.

There are a variety of musculoskeletal symptoms that can also mimic those caused by PAD. Orthopedic problems involving the knee and hip are most common. One entity in particular, trochanteric bursitis, often produces hip pain with walking. In many cases, trochanteric bursitis can be identified by aggressively palpating over the greater trochanter of the hip. When bursitis is present, this maneuver produces pain and tenderness. The patient may also tell you that he or she has difficulty lying on that hip at night, further raising the suspicion of a musculoskeletal abnormality.

When To Refer for Further Testing

The five most common indications for referral to a vascular laboratory for formal arterial testing include:

1. Screening: By definition, screening is performed on patients in whom there is no objective evidence of PAD, but in whom someone (typically the patient) has raised a concern about occult disease. As noted earlier, it is somewhat controversial (especially if referral to a vascular laboratory or for-profit screening service is involved). The cost effectiveness of screening will likely become clearer in the coming years.
2. Patients with findings (historical or on physical examination) suspicious for PAD: In this case, objective testing establishes or confirms the diagnosis of PAD. Because of its broad implications (for coronary, carotid, or other atherosclerotic problems), it is impor-

tant to obtain objective, high-quality information before labeling the patient as having PAD. This diagnosis will often lead to other tests for atherosclerosis involving the carotids or coronaries; these may be costly or even invasive, so objective documentation of PAD is justified before other tests are ordered (7).

3. Assessing the severity of disease in patients with known PAD: Often the diagnosis is not in question, but there is uncertainty regarding the severity of disease (8). In particular, it must be determined whether the PAD is severe enough to explain the patient's symptoms (9): for example, is the PAD so severe that it threatens the limb and therefore requires possible revascularization, even if the patient feels he or she can live with the symptoms? In situations where nonhealing leg wounds are present, tests for the adequacy of perfusion (such as transcutaneous oximetry) may be necessary to determine whether blood flow is adequate for healing purposes. Initial information about the feasibility of catheter-directed revascularization can be obtained from vascular laboratory studies. In each of these cases, and in many others, formal vascular laboratory testing is essential to determine the need for treatment and the therapeutic options that are likely available.

4. Serial studies: There may be concern about progression or regression of PAD over time. This is especially important when medical therapy has been instituted (including things like statins, exercise programs, etc.), and it is important to determine whether patients are objectively improving. Alternatively, the progression of disease over time may be important in deciding if (or when) to intervene with an invasive procedure. Referral to a noninvasive vascular laboratory enables this information to be obtained as often as necessary.

5. Risk of cardiac comorbidities: Many vascular laboratories offer treadmill testing as part of their evaluation for PAD. When this is performed, it may be possible to evaluate the patient's cardiac status in conjunction with the assessment of their PAD (by monitoring their symptoms, electrocardiogram, blood pressure, etc.). When cardiac symptoms or ECG changes are noted during low-level workloads associated with peripheral vascular laboratory exercise studies, referral to a cardiac facility for further workup is warranted (10).

REFERENCES

1. **Beckman JA, Creager MA.** The history and physical examination. In Vascular Medicine: A Companion to Braunwald's Heart Disease. Creager MA, Dzau VJ, Loscalzo J, eds. Elsevier, Inc; 2006:135-65.

2. **McDermott MM.** Leg symptoms in peripheral arterial disease: clinical characteristics and functional impairment. In Trends in Vascular Surgery. Pearce WH, Matsumura JS, Yao JS. Precept Press; 2002:13-23.

3. **Goldberg, Charlie.** A Practical Guide to Clinical Medicine: Examination of the Lower Extremities. University of California, San Diego, School of Medicine, 2005. http://medicine.ucsd.edu/clinicalmed/extremities.htm.

4. **Wennberg PW, Rooke TW.** Diagnosis and management of diseases of the peripheral arteries and veins. In Hurst's the Heart, 10th ed. Fuster V, Alexander RW, O'Rourke RA, eds. McGraw-Hill Companies, Inc; 2001:2421-41.

5. **Cooke JP, Creager MA, Osmundson PJ, Shepherd JT.** Sex differences in control of cutaneous blood flow. Circulation. 1990;82:1607-15.

6. **Doobay AV, Anand SS.** Sensitivity and specificity of the ankle-brachial index to predict future cardiovascular outcomes. Arterioscler Thrombos Vasc Biol. 2005;25:1463.

7. **McLafferty RB, Dunnington GL, Mattos MA, et al.** Factors affecting the diagnosis of peripheral vascular disease before vascular surgery referral. J Vasc Surg. 2000;31:870-9.

8. **Hicken GJ, Lossing AG, Ameli FM.** Assessment of generic health-related quality of life in patients with intermittent claudication. Eur J Vasc Endovasc Surg. 2000;20:336-41.

9. **Long J, Modrall JG, Parker BJ, et al.** Correlation between ankle-brachial index, symptoms, and health-related quality of life in patients with peripheral vascular disease. J Vasc Surg. 2004;39:723-7.

10. **Abir F, Kakisis I, Sumpio B.** Do vascular surgery patients need a cardiology work-up? A review of preoperative cardiac clearance guidelines in vascular surgery. Eur J Vasc Endovasc Surg. 2003;25:110-7.

KEY REFERENCES

Beckman JA, Creager MA. The history and physical examination. In Vascular Medicine: A Companion to Braunwald's Heart Disease. Creager MA, Dzau VJ, Loscalzo J, eds. Elsevier, Inc; 2006:135-65. *Although this chapter covers more than just the lower extremity arterial examination (it touches on venous exam, neck exam, examination for lymphedema, etc.) it is well written and extremely current. The photos and illustrations are excellent. The two authors are well-known for their ability to make "pithy" observations, even when the topic may be mundane.*

McDermott MM. Leg symptoms in peripheral arterial disease: clinical characteristics and functional impairment. In Trends in Vascular Surgery. Pearce WH, Matsumura JS, Yao JS. Precept Press; 2002:13-23. *This well-written overview gives excellent insight into the various questionnaires used to access the severity of claudication. It also highlights an important but frequently under-appreciated concept – PAD does not always produce typical claudication. Atypical or absent symptoms are not uncommon, even when the disease is significant.*

Goldberg, Charlie. A Practical Guide to Clinical Medicine: Examination of the Lower Extremities. University of California, San Diego, School of Medicine, 2005. http://medicine.ucsd.edu/clinicalmed/extremities.htm. *This is an excellent reference! It is well written, beautifully illustrated, and extremely effective at explaining the nuances of the vascular physical examination.*

Wennberg PW, Rooke TW. Diagnosis and management of diseases of the peripheral arteries and veins. In Hurst's the Heart, 10th ed. Fuster V, Alexander RW, O'Rourke RA, eds. McGraw-Hill Companies, Inc; 2001:2421-41. *This was included primarily to emphasize the pulse scoring system favored at our institution (and many others), but it also contains a reasonable overview of the history and physical exam for PAD.*

Cooke JP, Creager MA, Osmundson PJ, Shepherd JT. Sex differences in control of cutaneous blood flow. Circulation. 1990;82:1607-15. *Although this paper is 16-years-old, it is a "classic". The basic observation – that baseline skin blood flow in women is approxi-*

mately half that in men – provides a starting point for understanding benign sympto-matology such as "cold hands and feet" in otherwise normal individuals.

Doobay AV, Anand SS. Sensitivity and specificity of the ankle-brachial index to predict future cardiovascular outcomes. Arterioscler Thrombos Vasc Biol. 2005;25:1463. *A recent update of a well-recognized observation – the presence of PAD predicts an increased mortality. The paper is particularly valuable for the very complete list of references it provides.*

McLafferty RB, Dunnington GL, Mattos MA, et al. Factors affecting the diagnosis of periph-eral vascular disease before vascular surgery referral. J Vasc Surg. 2000;31:870-9. *This interesting paper demonstrates that general internists frequently fail to ask about clau-dication, check for pedal pulses, etc. When they are suspicious of vascular disease, they are likely to order noninvasive testing rather than refer patients directly to a vascular specialist.*

Hicken GJ, Lossing AG, Ameli FM. Assessment of generic health-related quality of life in pa-tients with intermittent claudication. Eur J Vasc Endovasc Surg. 2000;20:336-41. *This pa-per highlights the fact that surgeons and patients often do not agree on the severity of peripheral vascular disease. In particular, surgeons seem to have difficulty predicting the quality-of-life their patients are experiencing due to PAD. A low threshold for obtaining objective quality-of-life assessments is advocated.*

Long J, Modrall JG, Parker BJ, et al. Correlation between ankle-brachial index, symptoms, and health-related quality of life in patients with peripheral vascular disease. J Vasc Surg. 2004;39:723-7. *Another paper that raises concern about the physician's ability to predict the patient's quality of life using the ABI. The authors suggest that the patient's symptoms may be a better predictor than the objective test (ABI). Once again, the importance of a careful history is reinforced.*

Abir F, Kakisis I, Sumpio B. Do vascular surgery patients need a cardiology work-up? A review of preoperative cardiac clearance guidelines in vascular surgery. Eur J Vasc Endovasc Surg. 2003;25:110-7. *Articles arguing the need (or lack of need) for cardiac evaluation in patients with PAD are becoming a cottage industry. This paper reviews the large number of studies that have been performed in an attempt to clarify these muddy waters, and offers (what I consider to be) reasonable recommendations.*

Chapter 3

Noninvasive Evaluation of Peripheral Arterial Disease

OLUJIMI A. AJIJOLA, MD
MICHAEL R. JAFF, DO

1. What is the appropriate method of performing an ankle-brachial index?
2. What is the importance of non-compressible arteries found during the performance of the ankle-brachial index?
3. When should treadmill testing be performed, and how are the results interpreted?
4. What are the advantages and disadvantages of arterial duplex ultrasonography in providing a diagnosis of peripheral arterial disease?
5. What information is obtained via transcutaneous oximetry?

Peripheral arterial disease (PAD) remains an important cause of morbidity and mortality in today's society. Early and accurate diagnosis is a key strategy in managing this disease. Furthermore, routine surveillance and testing is very important in monitoring patients following therapy, either invasive or medical. The optimal properties of diagnostic tests for PAD include accurate, noninvasive, widely accessible, risk-free, inexpensive, and reliable examinations. A number of tests are currently available, each with its own advantages and disadvantages. This chapter will provide an overview and discuss the roles of noninvasive tests including: the ankle-brachial index (ABI), segmental limb pressures, Doppler waveforms, pulse-volume recordings, exercise testing, duplex ultrasonography, and transcutaneous oximetry.

The Role of the History and Physical Examination in the Diagnosis of Peripheral Arterial Disease

Performing an accurate and detailed history, combined with a thorough and comprehensive physical examination is critical in the diagnosis of PAD. Diagnostic testing without solid understanding of the symptoms and limitations due to PAD provides anatomic information alone, without considering the impact of PAD on quality of life, disability, and risk of limb loss. The severity of symptoms and physical examination findings of the patient largely determines the extent of testing required in each individual case. For example, the finding of a stenosis within the superficial femoral artery warrants atherosclerotic risk-factor intervention but not necessarily an invasive intervention.

Important elements of the history include the location of discomfort, quality of discomfort, conditions inducing and relieving symptoms, and the degree of functional limitation. Duration of symptoms and an assessment of the stability or worsening of the symptoms are critical. In a minority of patients, an appreciation of ischemic rest pain and non-healing limb ulcerations is important. This subset of patients may have critical limb ischemia, which usually requires prompt revascularization. Assessment of prior diagnostic tests and treatments are important to determine the duration, severity, and alternative therapies available. In every patient, determining the presence of co-morbid conditions such as diabetes mellitus, hyperlipidemia, tobacco use, hypertension, abdominal aortic aneurysms, and co-existing coronary, cerebrovascular, and renal artery disease is standard.

During the physical examination, auscultation for bruits over the cervical, carotid, abdomen/pelvic/flank, and femoral regions must be performed. The palpation of pulses of the carotid, brachial radial, femoral, popliteal, dorsalis pedis, and posterior tibial arteries is standard. Determining the presence of pallor on elevation and rubor with dependency, and searching for foot or digit ulcers, is routine. The findings of tinea pedis and callous formation, which may ultimately result in ischemic ulcerations in patients with advanced PAD, often with diabetes mellitus, is clinically important.

Ankle-Brachial Index

The ankle-brachial index (ABI) is a simple, accurate, reproducible, and inexpensive test that is commonly performed in the office setting. It involves the use of a standard sphygmomanometer, a hand-held continuous wave Doppler probe, and a small amount of acoustic coupling gel (Figure 3-1). The ABI is calculation of the ratio of the systolic blood pressure in the ankle (higher of the dorsalis pedis or posterior tibial artery) to that of the higher of the two brachial artery pressures. It is performed after a patient

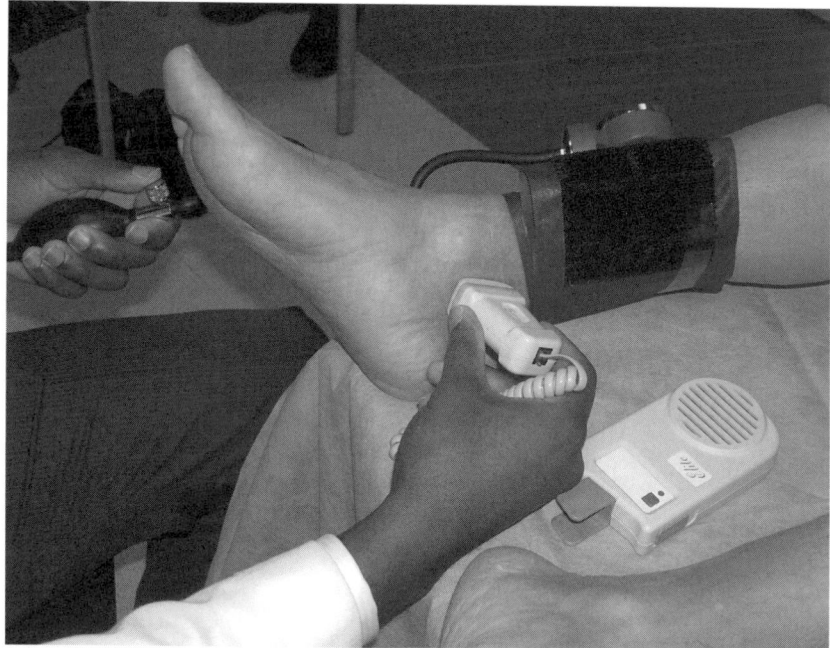

Figure 3-1. Demonstration of performance of ankle-brachial index by assessing the left posterior tibial artery systolic blood pressure.

has been resting supine for 5-10 minutes. Repeating it after the patient has performed exercise to the point of symptoms is the most accurate method of determining the physiologic severity of PAD. A decrease in the ABI following treadmill exercise or active pedal plantar flexion confirms the diagnosis of PAD and can be used to characterize the functional limitations of the patient.

In healthy individuals, the systolic blood pressure in the ankle generally exceeds the brachial systolic pressure by 10-15 mmHg due to the higher peripheral vascular resistance in the ankle vessels. The obtained ABI is interpreted according to Table 3-1.

Table 3-1.   Severity of PAD on Ankle-Brachial Index Results

ABI	Severity of PAD
≥1.30	Non-compressible vessel
1:00-1.29	Normal
0.91-0.99	Borderline/equivocal
0.41-0.90	Mild-to-moderate PAD
0.00-0.40	Severe PAD

A non-compressible vessel is one with significant medial artery calcification leading to falsely elevated pressures in the ankle arteries, thus leading to an ABI greater than 1.30. This is the primary limitation of the ABI, and is usually found in the elderly with diabetes mellitus, patients requiring hemodialysis for end-stage renal disease, and occasionally in patients with a history of chronic corticosteroid use. In this situation, patients must be referred to a formal vascular diagnostic laboratory for the assessment of digital arterial pressures.

The ABI correlates well with symptoms and functional limitation due to PAD and can predict the severity of PAD. Compared to angiography, the gold standard for the diagnosis of PAD, an ABI of equal to or less than 0.90, has a sensitivity and specificity of 95% and 100%, respectively, for detecting a stenotic lesion of 50% or greater in a limb (1,2). Further, the association between the ABI and cardiovascular morbidity and mortality, as well as reduction in limb function, has been demonstrated in numerous studies. In one cohort study of 154 patients with an ABI <0.90, the 5-year cumulative survival was 63% for those with resting ABI <0.50; 71% for those with ABI between 0.50 and 0.69; and 91% for those with ABI between 0.70 and 0.89 (3). These data were expanded upon in a study by Resnick and colleagues who demonstrated that the adjusted risk estimates for all-cause and cardiovascular disease mortality were similar in the low ABI group (1.69 and 2.52, respectively) and in patients with supranormal ABI (1.77 and 2.09, respectively) (2). Wang et al documented that both low-normal ABIs (0.91-0.99) and high ABIs (above 1.40) were associated with higher rates of lower-extremity symptoms than in patients with ABIs of 1.00-1.39 (3).

Recently, investigators have challenged the classic method of calculating the ABI, suggesting that the lower of the ankle pressures should be used as the numerator (4). In one study, investigators compared the high ankle pressure (HAP) methodology to their proposed low ankle pressure (LAP) method in 216 subjects who also underwent arterial duplex ultrasonography as the method of comparison. Using an ABI of <0.9 as the cut-off for significant stenosis, they found that the sensitivity of the HAP and LAP in detecting PAD was 89% and 68%, respectively, while the specificity was 93% and 99%, respectively. Current recommendations as defined in the American College of Cardiology/American Heart Association (ACC/AHA) Peripheral Arterial Disease Guidelines (5) and the TASC 2 guidelines (6) recommend performing resting ABIs in patients with exertional leg symptoms, critical limb ischemia, age 70 or older, or age 50-69 with a history of tobacco abuse and diabetes mellitus, where PAD is suspected. The American Diabetes Association formally recommends performing an ABI in all patients with diabetes mellitus under the age of 50 with history of tobacco abuse, hypertension, hyperlipidemia, or duration of diabetes greater than 10 years, and in all diabetic patients over the age of 50 (7).

Despite the overwhelming advantages of the ABI in the diagnosis of PAD and cardiovascular risk, its use is limited by the lack of reimbursement when performed in the office setting, and the perception of difficulty in completing the ABI (8).

When falsely elevated or normal ABIs are obtained in a patient in whom there is a high clinical index of suspicion of PAD, formal vascular laboratory testing is suggested. For those with ABI > 1.30, toe pressures and toe brachial indices (TBI) should be performed. This method is used to assess lower limb arterial perfusion, since digital arteries are less susceptible to arterial calcification (9). The TBI is performed using a blood pressure cuff designed for the toe, and a sophisticated photoplethysmograph to assess occlusion pressure in the toe. In general, the pressure in the great toe artery is lower than at the ankle, thus a TBI of <0.70 is considered diagnostic for PAD. The combination of digital pressures with pulse wave recordings obtained with plethysmography (10) may reflect the optimal noninvasive method of predicting the risk of limb loss or ischemic wound healing. Absolute toe pressures < 30 mmHg in association with diminished pulse wave amplitudes in the digit suggest inadequate arterial circulation to heal ischemic ulcerations, and often aids in the assessment of amputation levels (11,12).

In a study by Sahli et al, toe pressure (TP), ankle pressure (AP), toe-brachial index, and ankle-brachial index were studied in 437 subjects with Type 1 (DM 1) and Type 2 (DM 2) diabetes mellitus as well as normal controls. Variables were low in 24% of DM 1 and in 31% of DM 2 patients compared with only 6% of normal controls (13). Abnormally low TBI as well as low absolute TP were more common in the diabetic patients than low values of the ABI and absolute AP, confirming the incidence of arterial calcification in patients with diabetes mellitus.

In 136 men who underwent forefoot amputations, the predictive value of TP was demonstrated (14). In diabetic patients, when the TP was less than 40 mmHg, no healing occurred in the stump following digital amputation even if preceded by revascularization. However, when the TP was greater than 68 mmHg, or when there was an increase in TP of 30 mmHg or more following revascularization, all amputation stump sites healed.

Exercise Testing

The utility of the ABI is increased when combined with an exercise test. It is particularly useful in patients with suspected PAD but normal resting ABIs. It can directly help to assess whether symptoms of exertional limb discomfort are due to PAD or an alternate etiology. This examination is commonly performed in a vascular laboratory using a computerized programmable treadmill.

A baseline ABI is obtained prior to exercise. The patient is then placed on a treadmill at a constant speed (2.0 miles per hour) and constant grade (12%). Clinical trials of therapies for intermittent claudication commonly employ the Gardner treadmill protocol using a constant speed and variable grade beginning at 0% and increasing 2% every 2 minutes. The patient is exercised until symptoms occur, at which point the location and intensity of discomfort are recorded). Once maximal walking distance is reached, the protocol is discontinued. Associated symptoms such as exertional dyspnea, chest pain, and disequilibrium should be noted as well (15). Although some laboratories perform ABIs at 1-minute intervals following exercise until the baseline values are restored, one post-exercise measurement immediately following cessation of exercise is of equal validity. A normal exercise response represents stability or increase in the ABI after exercise (Figure 3-3).

Exercise testing is also useful the office setting. If there is concern regarding gait stability or cardiopulmonary reserve, or if a vascular laboratory is not readily available, the physician may use active pedal plantar flexion as a surrogate for treadmill testing. Patients are asked to hold on to a steady surface and rise up on their toes and then lower to a neutral position as rapidly as possible. At completion of this exercise, ABIs are again obtained. Active pedal plantar flexion correlates very well with treadmill exercise testing (16). A second major limitation of the ABI is that there is no ability to precisely determine the arterial segments affected by atherosclerosis and resulting in symptoms. One may only infer from an abnormal ABI that there is arterial disease at some level between the brachial and pedal arteries. Utilizing segmental limb pressures and pulse volume recordings in association with ABI, the physician may reliably predict the arterial segments involved.

Segmental Limb Pressures

With this technique, systolic blood pressures are obtained using a plethysmographic cuff at the upper thigh, lower thigh, upper calf (just below the level of the knee), ankle, metatarsal, and toe (Figure 3-2). The 3-cuff protocol excludes the lower thigh measurement. The four-cuff method, with two cuffs placed on the proximal and distal thigh, offers the advantage of allowing the interpreter to differentiate inflow vs. infrainguinal PAD. However, the proximal thigh cuff is often uncomfortable for patients, and depending on limb circumference, appropriate fit of the cuff may be impossible. These segmental systolic blood pressures are recorded and compared to determine the location of an arterial lesion. A gradient of 20 mmHg or greater from one segment to the next segment distal to it suggests peripheral arterial disease at the level just proximal to the distal cuff (17). For example, a systolic blood pressure of 120 mmHg taken at the upper calf, and one of 95 mmHg taken at the ankle indicate disease in tibioperoneal arteries. Segmental Limb Pressures (SLP) may be used alone, or (more commonly) performed in conjunction with pulse volume recordings (PVR). Comparison of pressure in one limb compared to the other is also useful for evaluating the presence of occlusive disease.

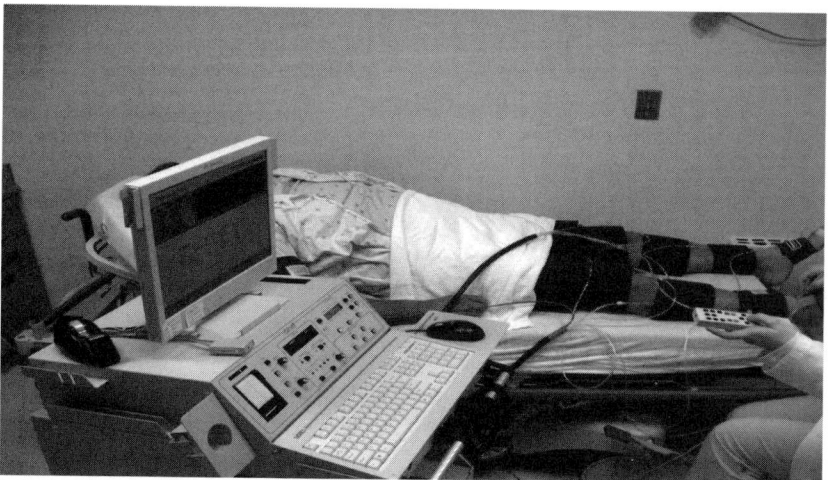

Figure 3-2. Example of patient positioning for performance of segmental limb pressures, pulse volume recordings and Doppler waveforms.

Exercise Pressure Measurement

	Rest	1	2	3	4	5	6	7	8	9	10
R Ankle (PT):	132	187									
L Ankle (PT):	136	176									
R Brachial:	113	139									
R ABI	1.17	1.35									
L ABI	1.20	1.27									

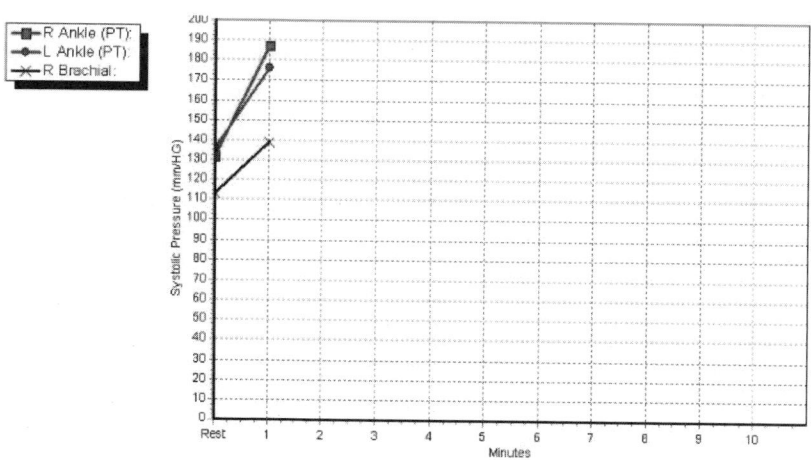

Figure 3-3. Normal treadmill exercise response with increase in post-exercise ankle arterial systolic blood pressures.

Pulse-Volume Recordings

Pulse-volume recordings (PVR) are plethysmographic tests designed to detect volume changes during arterial blood flow beneath the cuff (18). The contours of the waveform are evaluated to detect changes from normal, which provide additional information about the status of the lower-extremity arteries. It is a qualitative rather than a quantitative study, unlike the ABI. A normal waveform is similar to an intra-arterial waveform obtained during hemodynamic monitoring, and is notable for a steep upstroke, a sharp systolic peak, a narrow pulse waveform, a dicrotic notch, and a bowing downslope back to baseline (Figure 3-4). When PAD is present, blood flow across a stenosis increases, resulting in changes in the waveform morphology. Characteristic changes include delay of the upstroke, widening of the waveform with a rounded peak, loss of the dicrotic notch, and bowing of the downslope away from baseline (Figure 3-5). The PVR is less accurate in determining stenosis versus occlusion of the involved segment when

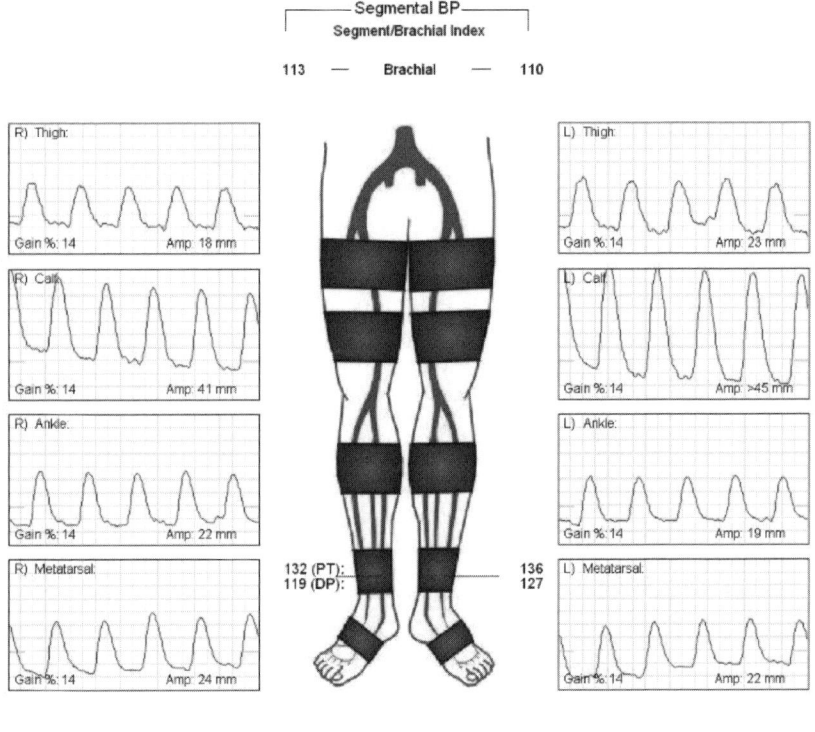

Figure 3-4. Normal segmental limb pressures, pulse volume recordings and ankle-brachial indices bilaterally at rest.

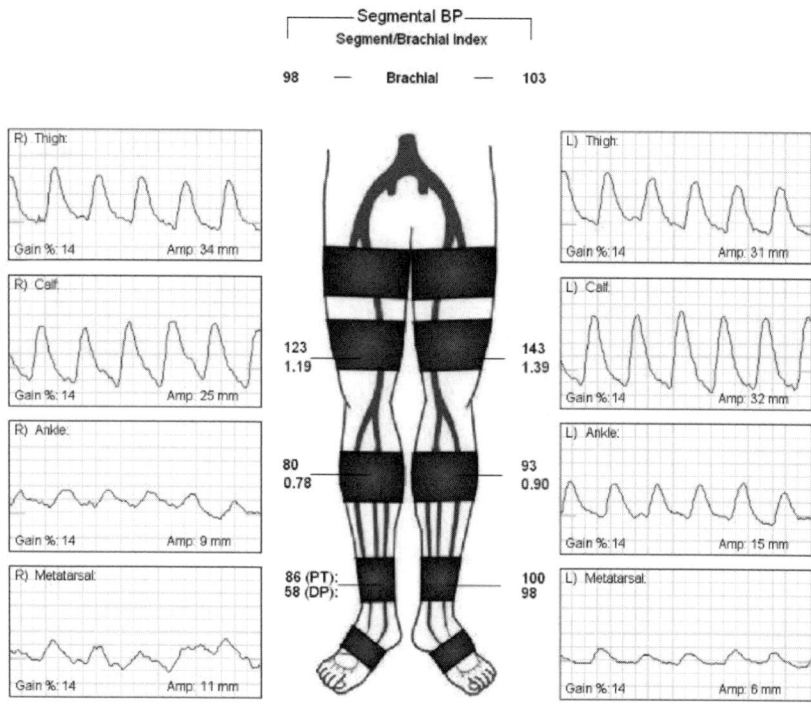

Figure 3-5. Abnormal segmental limb pressures, pulse volume recordings and ankle-brachial indices bilaterally at rest demonstrating infrapopliteal arterial disease bilaterally.

compared to direct imaging methods (i.e. duplex ultrasonography). However, PVRs are relatively simple to perform with less expensive equipment required than a modern color duplex ultrasound unit.

PVR waveforms are commonly obtained at the level of the metatarsal level by placing a cuff around the arch of the foot. A dampened or flat PVR at this region compared with those at the ankle indicate the presence of intrinsic small vessel disease, particularly if performed in a temperature-controlled room. This is important in evaluating the potential for wound healing of ulcers and after amputation of digits.

Arterial Duplex Ultrasonography

Ultrasonography refers to the use of sound waves to determine a variety of characteristics about the tissue or organ to which it is directed. The ultrasound wave penetrates tissues of varying densities and echogenic properties as it traverses its path, and is reflected back to the ultrasound probe (19).

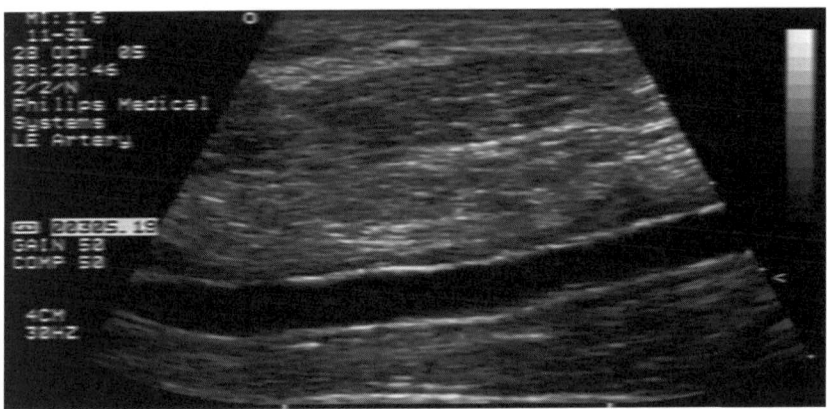

Figure 3-6.   Gray scale Doppler image of a stent in the superficial femoral artery.

Using Brightness mode technology (B-mode), many ultrasound machines can depict gray scale images in real-time; however, this depends on the frequency of the ultrasound waves and quality of images desired. High-frequency probes (10 MHz) provide great image resolution, but the beam is limited in depth penetration. Low-frequency probes (2 MHz) penetrate to visualize deeper structures, while image resolution is sacrificed (Figure 3-6). Duplex ultrasonography represents the addition of Doppler technology to B-mode imaging, allowing the visualization of flowing blood in arteries and veins. This technology also allows determination of blood velocity.

Assessment of arterial patency is performed by combining a number of variables including the known velocity of flowing blood, velocity of sound in tissue, the differences in the frequency of transmitted and reflected sound, and the cosine of the angle of the ultrasound beam to the direction of blood flow (the Doppler equation). Based on the velocity of blood in the region of interest, interpreters are able to determine degrees of stenosis.

Lower-extremity arterial duplex ultrasonography is widely accepted as a method of determining arterial stenoses or occlusions. Its sensitivity in detecting occlusions and stenoses is estimated to be 95% and 92%, with specificities of 99% and 97%, respectively (20). Vessels are typically examined anatomically in the sagittal plane, while Doppler velocities are obtained at a 60-degree Doppler angle. Vessels are generally classified according to the following scheme: normal, 1-19% stenosis, 20%-49% stenosis, 50%-99% stenosis, and occlusion. This degree of stenosis is determined by alterations in the Doppler waveform and peak systolic velocities. As an example, the peak systolic velocity must increase by 100% in comparison to the normal segment of artery proximal to the stenosis to be classified as a 50%-99% stenosis (21). The addition of color to the gray scale and Doppler image provides a rapid identification of areas of turbulence and stenosis (Figure 3-7).

Arterial duplex ultrasound is accurate, noninvasive, and relatively inexpensive, making it an indispensable test in the diagnosis of PAD. When per-

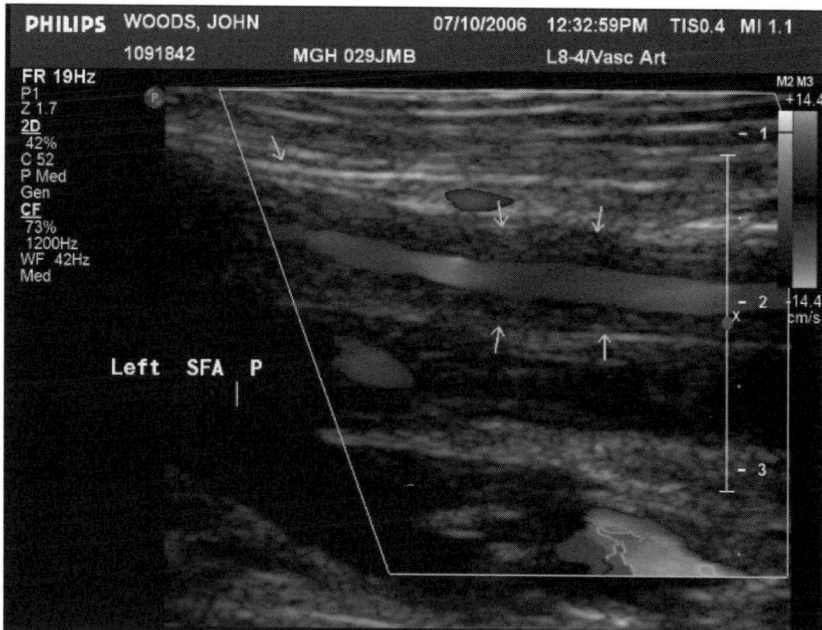

Figure 3-7.   Color Doppler image of diffuse in-stent restenosis of a stent in the superficial femoral artery.

formed at a center with expertise, management of severe lower-extremity ischemia can be based on duplex ultrasonography in most patients without negative effects on outcome (22). The strength of this modality in PAD may also extend beyond diagnosis in guiding angioplasty and stenting in patients with renal insufficiency in which the use of radiographic contrast is otherwise contraindicated (23,24).

Limitations of arterial duplex ultrasound in diagnosing arterial lesions have included tandem stenoses (25), tibial vessel imaging (26), imaging vessels near the knee (27) and difficulty imaging the inflow arteries (28). Further, a number of studies comparing ultrasound to contrast enhanced magnetic resonance angiography (MRA) argue that the sensitivity and specificity are greater with MRA than ultrasound in detecting hemodynamically significant stenotic lesions (27,29). It remains unknown whether this modality will overtake arterial duplex ultrasound as a diagnostic tool for PAD.

Transcutaneous Oximetry

Transcutaneous oximetry assesses microcirculatory perfusion of the skin, indicating the extent of PAD. It involves the use of heated electrodes, which generate a small amount of heat on the skin. This liquefies and disorganizes the solid crystalline structure of the stratum corneum, thus allowing for rapid gas diffusion, detected by a sensor placed on the skin. This sensor quantifies the cutaneous tension of oxygen ($TCPO_2$) and carbon dioxide ($TCPCO_2$) (30). It can be used to evaluate patients with vasospastic disease, as well as in planning revascularization. Many centers rely on transcutaneous oximetry to predict the likelihood of wound healing on the foot, as well as determining the level at which amputations may be successfully performed. Transcutaneous oximetry may differentiate well-perfused tissues from those with poor blood supply (31). In diabetics (and other diseases) where autonomic dysfunction alters the perfusion of the local tissues, assessment of blood flow alone is insufficient to predict wound healing. Zimny and colleagues confirmed the applicability of transcutaneous oximetry by detecting a difference in local oxygen pressure between diabetic feet with neuropathy but no ulceration compared to diabetic feet without neuropathy or ulceration, and feet of normal controls (32). This data demonstrates that $TCPO_2$ can be a powerful diagnostic tool in assessing peripheral arterial disease.

Although a clinically useful measure of local perfusion, the variability of $TCPO_2$ is a significant limitation in its applicability. Since $TCPO_2$ relies on several factors including the arterial pressure of oxygen and cardiac output, cardiopulmonary disease may significantly affect $TCPO_2$. Using a reference site, such as the chest wall $TCPO_2$, a presumably well-perfused site, can minimize this. This is called the Regional Perfusion Index (RPI). Use of the RPI reduces confounding variables in the clinical use of $TCPO_2$. Hauser et al demonstrated this in their study using the RPI to quantify tissue perfusion in PAD (30). They demonstrated variability in the systemic oxygen delivery and its affect on $TCPO_2$. The use of the RPI resulted in an accurate and useful objective measure of local perfusion (30). Other obstacles preventing the widespread use of $TCPO_2$ include the need for a temperature controlled room, an examining table which promotes ideal positioning of the limb, requirements to allow the patient to rest quietly for 45 minutes, and a multi-chamber oximeter, which is quite expensive.

Future Noninvasive Testing for Peripheral Arterial Disease

There are a number of emerging modalities that will likely improve our ability to noninvasively diagnose PAD. These include magnetic resonance flowmetry, laser Doppler Flowmetry, and contrast-enhanced duplex ultrasonography. Others, such as magnetic resonance arteriography (MRA), computerized tomographic arteriography (CTA), and positron emission tomography will be covered in subsequent chapters of this text. These modalities offer additional information but will not supplant the use of the ABI, segmental pressures, PVRs and exercise treadmill testing. Magnetic resonance flowmetry employs the use of a cylindrical crossed-coil nuclear magnetic resonance flowmeter that is able to measure arterial blood flow through human arteries (33). It is noninvasive, does not require skin contact, and has the advantage of accurate measurement unimpaired by materials overlying the body surface in as little as 2 minutes. It is as yet not widely used, and its role in testing and diagnosis of PAD is unknown.

Conclusion

Peripheral arterial disease represents a significant cause of morbidity and mortality and accounts for a significant portion of healthcare expenditure. Early, accurate, noninvasive, reliable and inexpensive approaches to the diagnosis of PAD is a key strategy preventing major changes in quality of life, limb loss, myocardial infarction, stroke and death. There are several noninvasive tests currently available.

Guidelines from the ACC/AHA provide a straightforward approach to the evaluation and diagnosis of PAD. For asymptomatic patients at high risk for PAD, the ankle-brachial index is the preferred initial test. In those patients with symptomatic PAD, the ABI, PVR with SLP, and treadmill exercise testing are employed. If pseudoclaudication is suspected, an ABI with exercise is the preferred modality.

Lastly, when considering revascularization in patients with lifestyle-interfering intermittent claudication, and critical limb ischemia, direct imaging with arterial duplex ultrasonography is reasonable.

In patients with non-healing ulcerations or who require amputation, the use of digital pressures, waveforms, and transcutaneous oximetry may be helpful.

REFERENCES

1. Sikkink CJ, van Asten WN, van't Hof MA, et al. Decreased ankle/brachial indices in relation to morbidity and mortality in patients with peripheral arterial disease. Vasc Med. 1997; 2:169-73.
2. Resnick HE, Lindsay RS, McDermott MM, et al. Relationship of high and low ankle brachial index to all-cause and cardiovascular disease mortality: the Strong Heart Study. Circulation. 2004;109:733-9.
3. Wang JC, Criqui MH, Denenberg JO, et al. Exertional leg pain in patients with and without peripheral arterial disease. Circulation. 2005;112:3501-8.
4. Schroder F, Diehm N, Kareem S, et al. A modified calculation of ankle-brachial pressure index is far more sensitive in the detection of peripheral arterial disease. J Vasc Surg. 2006;44:531-6.
5. Hirsch AT, Haskal ZJ, Hertzer NR, et al. ACC/AHA 2005 guidelines for the management of patients with peripheral arterial disease (lower-extremity, renal, mesenteric, and abdominal aortic):executive summary. J Am Coll Cardiol. 2006;47:1239-312.
6. Norgren L, Hiatt WR, Dormandy JA, et al. Inter-Society consensus for the management of peripheral arterial disease (TASC II). J Vasc Surg. 2007;(Suppl)45:S5A-S67A.
7. American Diabetes Association. Peripheral arterial disease in people with diabetes. Diabetes Care. 2003;26:3333-41.

8. Mohler ER, et al. Utility and barriers to performance of the ankle-brachial index in primary care practice, Vascular Medicine 2004.

9. Brooks B, Dean R, Patel S, Wu B, Molyneaux L, Yue DK. TBI or not TBI: that is the question. Is it better to measure toe pressure than ankle pressure in diabetic patients? Diabet Med. 2001;18:528-32.

10. van den Broek TA, Dwars BJ, Rauwerda JA, Bakker FC. Plethysmographic selection of amputation level in peripheral vascular disease. J Vasc Surg. 1998;8:10-13.

11. Gensler SW, Haimovici H, Hoffert P, et al. Study of vascular lesions in diabetic, nondiabetic patients. Arch Surg. 1965;617-22.

12. Carter SA, Tate RB. Value of toe pulse waves in addition to systolic pressures in the assessment of the severity of peripheral arterial disease and critical limb ischemia. J Vasc Surg. 1996;24:258-65.

13. Sahli D, Eliasson B, Svensson M, et al. Assessment of toe blood pressure is an effective screening method to identify diabetes patients with lower-extremity arterial disease. Angiology. 2004;55:641-51.

14. Vitti MJ, Robinson DV, Hauer-Jensen M, et al. Wound healing in forefoot amputations: the predictive value of toe pressure. Ann Vasc Surg. 1994;8:99-106.

15. Feinglass J, McCarthy WJ, Slavensky R, et al. Effect of lower-extremity blood pressure on physical functioning in patients who have intermittent claudication. J Vasc Surg. 1996;24:503-12.

16. McPhail IR, Spittell PC, Weston SA, Bailey KR. Intermittent claudication: an objective office based assessment. J Am Coll Cardiol. 2001;37:1381-5.

17. Strandness DE. Noninvasive vascular laboratory and vascular imaging. In: Young JR, Olin JW, Bartholomew JR, eds. Peripheral Vascular Diseases, 2nd ed. Philadelphia: Mosby Publishing Company; 1996:33-64.

18. MacDonald NR. Pulse volume plethysmography. J Vasc Tech. 1994;18:241-8.

19. Stewart JH, Grubb M. Understanding vascular ultrasonography. Mayo Clin Proc. 1992;67:1186-96.

20. Whelan JF, Barry MH, Moir JD. Color flow Doppler ultrasonography: comparison with peripheral arteriography for the investigation of peripheral vascular disease. J Clin Ultrasound. 1992;20:369-74.

21. Kohler TR, Nance DR, Cramer MM, et al. Duplex scanning for diagnosis of aortoiliac and femoropopliteal disease: a prospective study. Circulation. 1987;76:1074-80.

22. Koelemay MJ, Legemate DA, de Vos H, et al. Duplex scanning allows selective use of arteriography in the management of patients with severe lower leg arterial disease. J Vasc Surg. 2001;34:661-7

23. Ascher E, Marks NA, Schutzer RW, Hingorani AP. Duplex-guided balloon angioplasty and stenting for femoropopliteal arterial occlusive disease: an alternative in patients with renal insufficiency. J Vasc Surg. 2005;42:1108-13.

24. Ascher E, Marks NA, Hingorani AP, et al. Duplex-guided balloon angioplasty and subintimal dissection of infrapopliteal arteries: early results with a new approach to avoid radiation exposure and contrast material. J Vasc Surg. 2005;42:1114-21.

25. Allard L, Cloutier G, Durand LG, et al. Limitations of ultrasonic duplex scanning for diagnosing lower limb arterial stenoses in the presence of adjacent segment disease. J Vasc Surg. 1994;19:650-7.

26. Larch E, Minar E, Ahmadi R, et al. Value of color duplex sonography for evaluation of tibioperoneal arteries in patients with femoropopliteal obstruction: a prospective comparison with anterograde intraarterial digital subtraction angiography. J Vasc Surg. 1997;25:629-36.

27. Gjonnaess E, Morken B, Sandback G, et al. Gadolinium-enhanced magnetic resonance angiography, colour duplex and digital subtraction angiography of the lower limb arteries from the aorta to the tibio-peroneal trunk in patients with intermittent cludication. Eur J Vasc Endovasc Surg. 2006;31:53-8.

28. Lewis WA, Bray AE, Harrison CL, et al. A comparison of common femoral waveform analysis with aorto-iliac duplex scanning in assessment of aorto-iliac disease. J Vasc Tech. 1994;18:337-44.
29. Leinert T, Kessels AG, Nelemans PJ, et al. Peripheral arterial disease: comparison of color duplex US and contrast-enhanced MR angiography for diagnosis. Radiology. 2005;235:699-708.
30. Hauser CJ, Shoemaker WC. Use of a transcutaneous PO_2 Regional Perfusion Index to quantify tissue perfusion in peripheral vascular disease. Ann Surg. 1983;197:337-43.
31. Halperin JL. Evaluation of patients with peripheral vascular disease. Thrombosis Res. 2002;106:V303-11.
32. Zimny S, Dessel F, Ehren M, et al. Early detection of microcirculatory impairment in diabetic patients with foot at risk. Diabetes Care. 2001;24:1810-14.
33. Waveforms correlate with arteriography. J Vasc Tech. 1993;17(3/4):77.

KEY REFERENCES

American Diabetes Association. Peripheral arterial disease in people with diabetes. Diabetes Care 2003;26:3333-3341. This is a consensus document describing the evaluation and management of patients with peripheral arterial disease who have diabetes mellitus.

Norgren L, Hiatt WR, Dormandy JA, et al. Inter-Society consensus for the management of peripheral arterial disease (TASC II). J Vasc Surg 2007;45 (Suppl):S5A-S67A. This international document represents an exhaustive analysis of the current epidemiology, diagnosis, and management strategies for peripheral arterial disease of the lower-extremity arteries.

Hirsch AT, Haskal ZJ, Hertzer NR, et al. ACC/AHA 2005 guidelines for the management of patients with peripheral arterial disease (lower-extremity, renal, mesenteric, and abdominal aortic):executive summary. J Am Coll Cardiol 2006;47:1239-1312. This multisocietal US consensus document analyzes all aspects of peripheral arterial disease, including lower-extremity disease.

McPhail IR, Spittell PC, Weston SA, and Bailey KR. Intermittent claudication: an objective office based assessment. J Am Coll Cardiol 2001 Apr;37(5):1381-5. This study demonstrates the utility of active pedal plantarflexion as a surrogate for treadmill testing in the office setting.

Koelemay MJ, Legemate DA, de Vos H, van Gurp AJ, Balm R, Reekers JA, and Jacobs MJ. Duplex scanning allows selective use of arteriography in the management of patients with severe lower leg arterial disease. J Vasc Surg 2001 Oct;34(4):661-7. This study demonstrates the utility of arterial duplex ultrasonography as a method of diagnosis of peripheral arterial disease.

Leinert T, Kessels AG, Nelemans PJ, Vashbinder GB, et al. Peripheral arterial disease: comparison of color duplex US and contrast-enhanced MR angiography for diagnosis. Radiology 2005 May; 235(2):699-708. Duplex ultrasonography compares quite well with magnetic resonance arteriography in the diagnosis of peripheral arterial disease.

Chapter 4

Magnetic Resonance, Computed Tomographic and Angiographic Imaging of Peripheral Arterial Disease

COREY K. GOLDMAN, MD, PhD
YUNG-WEI CHI, DO

1. What are the advantages/disadvantages of magnetic resonance arteriography?
2. What are the advantages/disadvantages of computed tomography?
3. What are the complications and risks of magnetic resonance arteriography and computed tomography?
4. When should I refer my patients for catheter-based arteriography?
5. What is the diagnostic algorithm for peripheral arterial disease?

The most significant advances in the evaluation of peripheral arterial disease (PAD) have involved the use of computerized tomographic angiography (CTA) and magnetic resonance angiography (MRA) with high-resolution imaging of vascular anatomy. This chapter describes key aspects and indications of both noninvasive and invasive angiography relevant to clinical management of PAD (1).

In the past, physiological testing as assessed with the ankle brachial index (ABI) and duplex ultrasound represented the standard noninvasive evaluation prior to referral for invasive angiography. With the widespread availability of CTA and MRA, anatomic definition of PAD can be achieved noninvasively and complements physiological testing in stratification of patients into available therapeutic strategies of surgical, endovascular, and medical options. In general, referral to invasive angiography of the extremities is limited to patients with anticipated endovascular or surgical intervention. MRA and CTA have become the more advanced forms of noninvasive angiography and are now recognized as appropriate tools to define and evaluate the extent of PAD as defined in a multidisciplinary position statement (2). In addition to the vessel topography information afforded by standard invasive angiography, both MRA and CTA also allow depiction of the lumen in a 3-dimensional representation. Additionally, CTA and MRA permit visualization of plaque, thrombus, vessel-wall thickening, aneurysms, extrinsic compression, dissections, and intramural hematomas, conditions that are not well depicted in standard angiography. Finally, both modalities provide imaging of the soft tissues and organs surrounding the vascular structures.

Magnetic Resonance Angiography

General Magnetic Resonance Principles

MRA has been available as a mean of assessing lower-extremity arteries since the 1990s. Contemporary MRA magnets with >1 Telsa strength are able to produce highly diagnostic studies even in the infrapopliteal segments. Images obtained using MR are related to altering the magnetic fields in regions containing nuclei with unpaired spin and is attributable predominantly to hydrogen nuclei in the human body. A magnetic field (B0) aligns the nuclei and a net angular rotation (precession) is generated. At a specified radiofrequency (RF) during MR imaging (MRI), H_1 atoms are excited. The return of the hydrogen nucleus to the basal state following the cessation of the RF pulse is called relaxation. The time required for the longitudinal vector to return to its value prior to the RF pulse is called longitudinal relaxation time (T1). The time required for return to the spin transverse to the magnetic field is termed (T2). For routine MRI, the relaxation times allow characterization of specific tissues. Both T1 and T2 depend on the physical and chemical magnetic enviroment and are different for different tissues. Tissues with a short T1 appear bright, whereas those with a long T1 appear dark. Tissues with a long T2 appear bright, and short T2 appear dark. Because the contents of vascular structures (blood) move fast distally from the time of excitation to the time of relaxation, the appearance of vessels in standard MR protocols is black or devoid of signal, and alternative techniques are employed for characterizing vasculature. The initial report demonstrating the utility of phase-contrast MRI for angiography was published in 1985 (3). This technique has not gained widespead use, and subsequent techniques have been devised to reveal the location of moving blood within MRI and to produce an image that accurately depicts vasculature (4).

Two-dimensional time of flight (2-D TOF) is a technique used for arterial imaging and does not require the use of intravascular contrast administration. Unlike other vascular imaging techniques, non-contrast MRA displays blood flow and not the vessel itself. In the 1990s and early 2000s, 2-D TOF has represented the standard of care for lower-extremity MRA. This technique is gradually being replaced by contrast-enhanced 3-dimensional MRA (CE-MRA) because of increased accuracy (Figure 4-1). In several clinical trials, CE-MRA was superior to 2D-TOF but requires more operator time due to arterial timing of gadolinium-contrast injection.

Sensitivity and Specificity

The accuracy of MRA for the anatomic definition of PAD is based on the technique employed for image acquisition as well as the experience of the

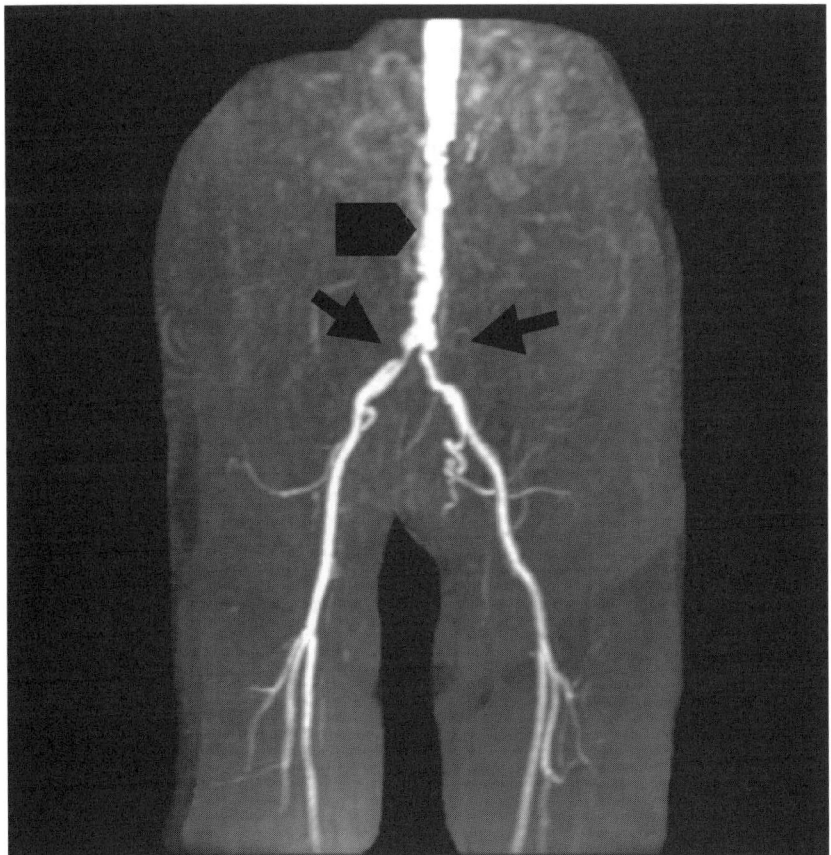

Figure 4-1. MRA of abdomen and lower extremity. Black arrows point to the severe common iliac artery ostial stenosis and black arrowhead points to atherosclerotic aorta.

imaging center with MRA (4). CE-MRA is considered standard practice for MRA and serves as a reference point for the accuracy of other techniques. In experienced hands, CE-MRA has sensitivity over 90% and specificity over 95% for the anatomic definition of PAD as compared to standard digital subtraction angiography (DSA) (5). 2D TOF MRA, which has commonly exaggerated the severity of stenoses, does not employ contrast and has lower accuracy. Newer techniques, including time-resolved imaging and dedicated lower-extremity magnetic coils are now being investigated.

Advantages

Contrast
Until recently, MRA distinguished itself from other imaging modalities on the basis of gadolinium-based contrast safety. The average circulation of time of gadolinium is 5 minutes, whereas investigational agents such as MS-325 that are bound to albumin can circulate up to 1 hour. However, although uncommon, there is recent recognition of an association between gadolinium use for MR and the development of nephrogenic systemic fibrosis in patients with moderate or severe renal insufficiency (6). Additionally there are some reports documenting rare worsening of severe renal insufficiency from gadolinium based-contrast (7). It is not known whether hydration has an impact on these adverse events. In patients with normal renal function, gadolinium-based contrast agents are very well tolerated. One technique under investigation to evaluate blood flow and tissue perfusion is the so-called "double-spin labeling." In this technique, arterial water is magnetically labeled, and local water diffusion allows evaluation of local tissue perfusion. This technique may be useful for differentiating flow-limiting lesions from incidental plaque.

Anatomy
Anatomic definition of abnormal arterial walls accompanying aneurysms or giant cell arteritis is exceptional in MRA combined with MRI and cannot be achieved with standard invasive angiography. Furthermore, the 3-dimensional relation of vessels to surrounding anatomy can be examined using computer-aided reconstruction after the diagnostic test is completed, whereas standard angiogram and duplex ultrasound have defined views taken during the study that are not readily manipulated once the study is complete. Lastly, MRA can also identify areas of active inflammation that may not be characterized by other vascular-imaging modalities.

Radiation
The images obtained using MRA are obtained by subjecting tissues to strong magnetic fields estimated at 60,000 times the magnetic field on earth. Despite this, there are no known morbidities directly attributable to fields with this intensity. Thus, the lack of ionizing irradiation represents a major positive attribute for MRA relative to CTA and standard angiogram.

Definition of Plaque

Atherosclerotic plaques are of heterogeneous composition. Plaque location, geometry, and composition are all useful indicators of vulnerability. In particular, the presence of a large extracellular lipid core, thin fibrous cap, and inflammatory cell infiltrate indicates plaques at risk. MR characterizes plaque on the basis of the biophysical and biochemical properties of its different components. Compared to the fibrous cap or media, the atheromatous core appears dark compared with the adjacent cap and media, which appear bright on T2-weighted images. Calcified areas of plaque do not generate appreciable signal because of the low water content and appear as areas of low signal (black) on T1-weighted images (Figure 4-2). Gadolinium chelates enhance T1 relaxation and therefore increase contrast enhancement on T1 image. This has been used to improve blood-tissue contrast, including neovascularization of plaque, which has been reported to further distinguish the necrotic core and fibrous cap and to highlight vulnerable plaque (8).

Disadvantages

Technical Factors

While all vascular imaging is dependent upon the operator, MRA has multiple technical parameters that vary with each particular center. Thus, image quality may be variable from center to center.

Claustrophobia

Moderate-to-severe anxiety has been documented in 37% of patients undergoing MRI, and 5%-10% of patients have symptoms that interfere with performing the study. There are some reports demonstrating the efficacy of both behavioral therapy and benzodiazepines to increase MRI study tolerability. Caution needs to be taken when outpatient pharmacological interventions leading to sedation are pursued because patients may not

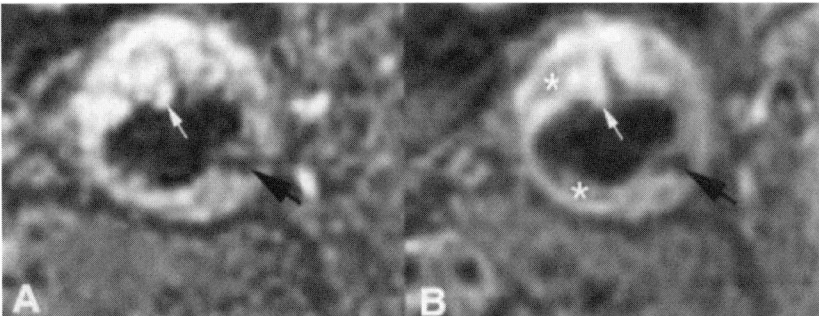

Figure 4-2.   MR characterization of plaque components. A, T1W image; B, T2W image. A complex lesion is detected with a fissure at 12 o'clock. Black arrows indicate calcium; asterisk, lipid deposits; and white arrows, thrombus.

recognize the need to avoid driving after the study, and there is a recent litigated case of a motor vehicle accident occurring after a patient was prescribed outpatient sedation in preparation for an MRI. Some centers do have the capability to perform monitored sedation and anesthesia during MRA when indicated.

Metallic Objects

Patients should be carefully screened for any implants as well as the date of implantation. While contemporary implants such as stents, hip prostheses, mechanical heart valves, oral implants, braces, or retainers are not directly affected by MRI because of the absence of ferromagnetic material, patients with either pacemakers or automatic defibrillators should not be referred for MRA. Patients with intracranial aneurysm clips should be managed on an individual basis and should not be sent to MRI unless the exact nature of the clip is determined to be MRI-safe. Specific identification of the manufacturer and type of aneurysm clip should be identified if the patient is to be sent for MRI.

Increasingly, vascular stents are being employed in the lower extremities for PAD. While stents are not a contraindication to MRA, image quality is severely impaired, and the resulting images do not provide useful information about the patency of stents.

Magnetic Resonance Angiography Costs

Although cost may differ due to regional and insurance payor differences, in general a CE-MRA costs about two times more than CTA, three to four times more than duplex ultrasound, and half the cost of contrast angiography.

Weight

MRA cannot be performed in the severely obese patient (weight >400 lbs).

Indications

MRA is used to determine the extent of PAD in anticipation of percutaneous or surgical intervention in patients with lifestyle-limiting claudication, ischemic rest pain, non-healing ischemic ulcerations, gangrene, and unexplained or recurrent atheroembolism. More recently, MRA has been indicated as possible first-line diagnostic mode for the investigation of PAD (Table 4-1).

Other indications may include evaluation of inflammatory and aneurysmal diseases, thromboembolic disease, vascular injury, arteritis, arterial dissection, spontaneous and iatrogenic, venous diseases, congenital vascular abnormalities, and dynamic compression of an entrapped popliteal artery.

Table 4-1.   Indications and Contraindications for Vascular Imaging Studies

	MRA	CTA	DSA
Indications	• Initial assessment of PAD • Lifestyle limiting claudication • Ischemic rest pain • Ischemic ulceration	• Initial assessment of PAD • Lifestyle-limiting claudication • Ischemic rest pain • Ischemic ulceration	• Lifestyle-limiting claudication • Ischemic rest pain • Ischemic ulceration
Contraindications	• Moderate and severe renal insufficiency (nephrogenic systemic fibrosis) • Claustrophobia • Pacemaker • Automatic defibrillator • Aneurysm clips (case by case basis)	• Severe renal insufficiency • Severe contrast • Allergy	• Severe renal insufficiency • Severe contrast • Allergy • Type IV Ehrlos • Danlos syndrome

Contraindications

As stated previously, patients with a pacemaker, an implantable defibrillator, or one who is severely claustrophobic should not be referred for MRA.

Patient Preparation

Patients with a history of claustrophobia should be identified prior to referral for MRI and, as previously noted, consideration for alternative study or sedation should be considered. Prior to entry into the MRI imaging suite, all paramagnetic objects such as jewelry and belt buckles must be removed. Patients should be informed that they will likely undergo placement of an IV for injection of gadolinium/contrast. Many MRI magnets are quite loud, and patients will frequently be given headphones or earplugs for the study. Study time ranges from 30 minutes to 75 minutes, depending upon the type of study performed.

Computed Tomographic Angiography

CTA has shown great potential as a noninvasive imaging modality of the lower-extremity arteries. CTA is frequently used to generate 3-dimensional images of the arteries that allow more intuitive interpretation of lower-extremity arterial anatomy and permits clinical decision making that previously required invasive angiography. An additional strength of CTA relates to the fine detail that can be achieved when examining reconstructed planar images.

General Computed Tomography Angiography Principles

The basic principle of CTA is similar to conventional X-ray. Initially, X-rays are generated by an "X-ray tube" and directed through the body part being imaged. The incident X-rays are attenuated (weakened) based on the density of the structures passed. The transmitted X-ray energy is captured by a scintillation crystal and emits light that is captured by detectors that are situated in rows. The analog signal of light is converted to a digital representation and stored in the computer memory for computer-aided reconstruction. Image reconstruction is based on mathematical algorithms that incorporate the speed of the X-ray source rotation relative to the motion of the patient table and the geometry of the X-ray beam spread prior to reaching the detectors. While first-generation CT scanners captured discrete data sets obtained through a single cross-section of the body, spiral scanning detectors capture a data set corresponding to the spiral path simulated as the body steadily traverses the rotating X-ray source. In the case of multi-detector CTA, multiple intersecting spiral datasets are generated, and image reconstruction takes place based on the configuration and width of the detectors.

Although CTA imaging of the lower-extremity arteries was initially attempted using a single-detector row scanner, it was not until the introduction of multiple-detector row CT (MDCT) in the 1990s that imaging of the entire inflow and runoff became possible. The visualization of small branches and large vascular territories with single-detector row CT (SDCT) angiography, such as lower extremities, has been limited due to the limited volume coverage and spatial resolution. Early studies correctly depicted segmental occlusions and significant stenoses, with sensitivities ranging between 91% and 94%, and specificities of 93%-97% (9,10). Over the past decade, advancement of CTA technology has enabled better image resolution and shorter acquisition time, utlizing increasing row detectors from 4- to 8- to 16-channel detectors, and now 64-channel detector CT is commercially available with submillimeter acquisition of the entire peripheral arterial tree. Resolution enhancement by muti-detector CTA is a necessity, especially for visualizing distal arteries such as the pedal and crural branches (Figure 4-3).

Multi-detector CT angiography provides three major advantages over single-detector CT angiography: shorter scanning durations associated with improved contrast-medium efficiency, thinner sections of entire anatomic territories within a breath hold, and greater longitudinal coverage. In recent years, a complete acquisition of lower-extremity inflow and run-off has become a real possibility with MDCT angiography (Figures 4-4, 4-5). MDCT angiography not only differentiates between high-grade and low-grade

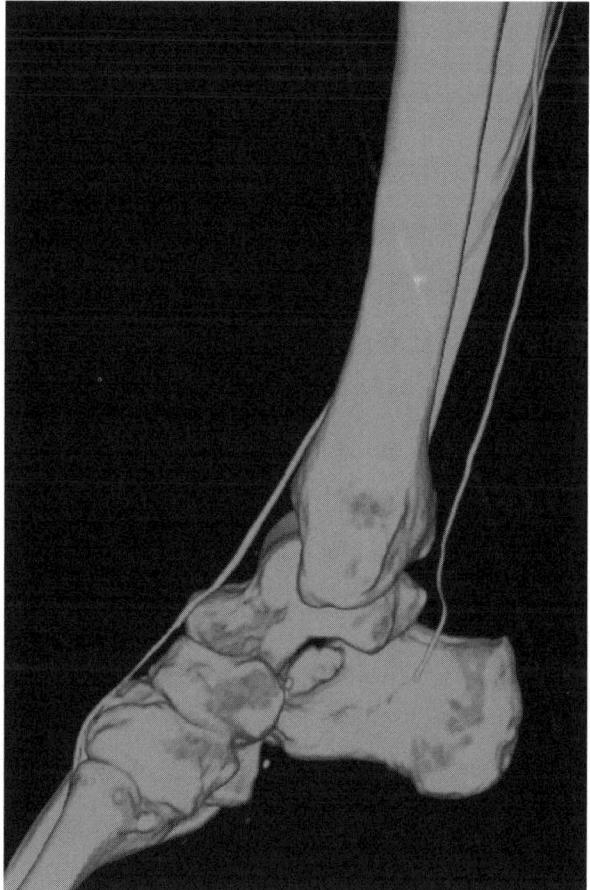

Figure 4-3. Pedal branch on CTA

stenoses in peripheral vasculature, but also improves characterization of the lesion, differentiating atheromatous from thrombotic occlusions.

Rubin et al (11) compared the utility of 4- versus 1-channel CT for evaluation of peripheral arteries. Compared to SDCT, MDCT angiography with 4-slice scanner was 2.6 times faster, scanning efficiency was 4.1 times greater, contrast efficiency was 2.5 times greater, dose of contrast material was nearly 47% less (97 vs. 232 mL) without a significant change in aortic enhancement, and sections were 40% thinner (3.2 mm vs. 5.3 mm), despite a 59% shorter scanning duration (22 seconds vs. 56 seconds).

Several studies of MDCT angiography demonstrated sensitivies and specificities of well over 90% as compared to DSA. These studies not only revealed very high concordance between DSA and CTA, but also showed that CTA may demonstrate vessels not visualized with DSA. Rubin (12) revealed a 100% concordance of revealing stenoses at direct comparison in

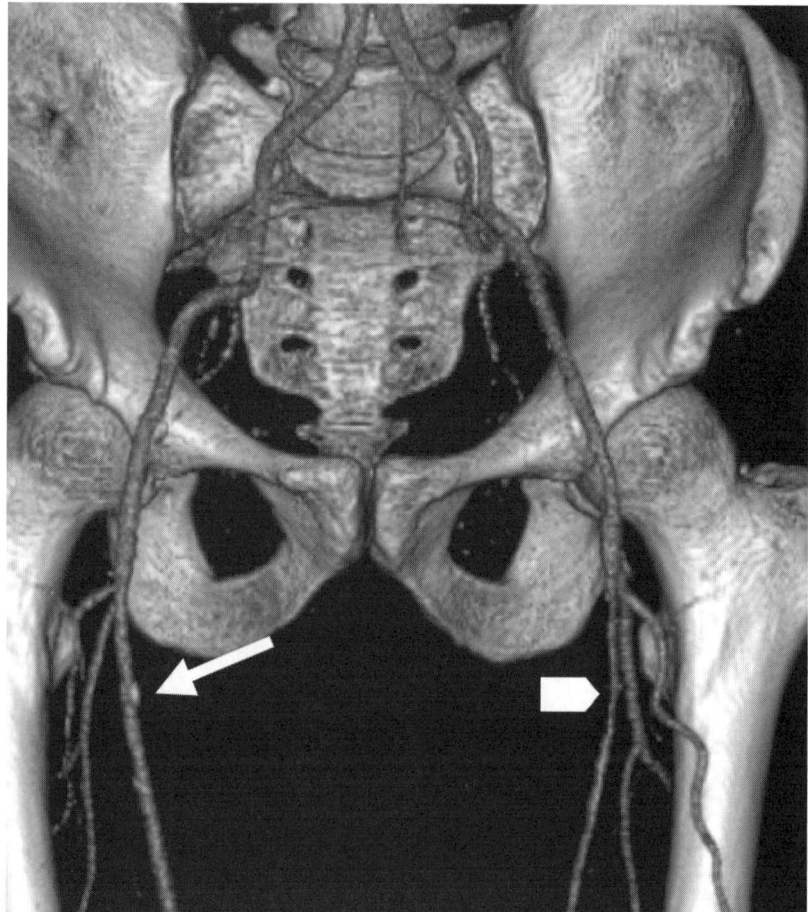

Figure 4-4. CTA of lower extremity vessels. Arrow points to a patent right superficial femoral artery associated with local calcium in the vessels wall. Arrowhead points to a stenotic left superficial femoral artery.

segments shown on both MDCT angiography and conventional angiography. MDCT angiography was also able to depict 26 arterial segments that were not visualized with DSA distal to more occluded segments. Martin et al (13) demonstrated sensitivity and specificity of MDCT angiography at 92% and 97%, respectively. In this study, multi-detector CTA again showed 110 more arterial segments than DSA; 90% were in the calves. In a landmark study, Willmann et al (14) compared the accuracy of 4-slice MDCT angiography with contrast-enhanced 3-D MRA for assessment of the aortoiliac segments in 46 consecutive patients (mean age: 68 years; 39 men) using DSA as the standard of reference. MDCT angiography revealed a sensitivity of 91% and a specificity of 99%, similar to MRA (MRA had a sensitivity and specificity of 92% and 99%, respectively).

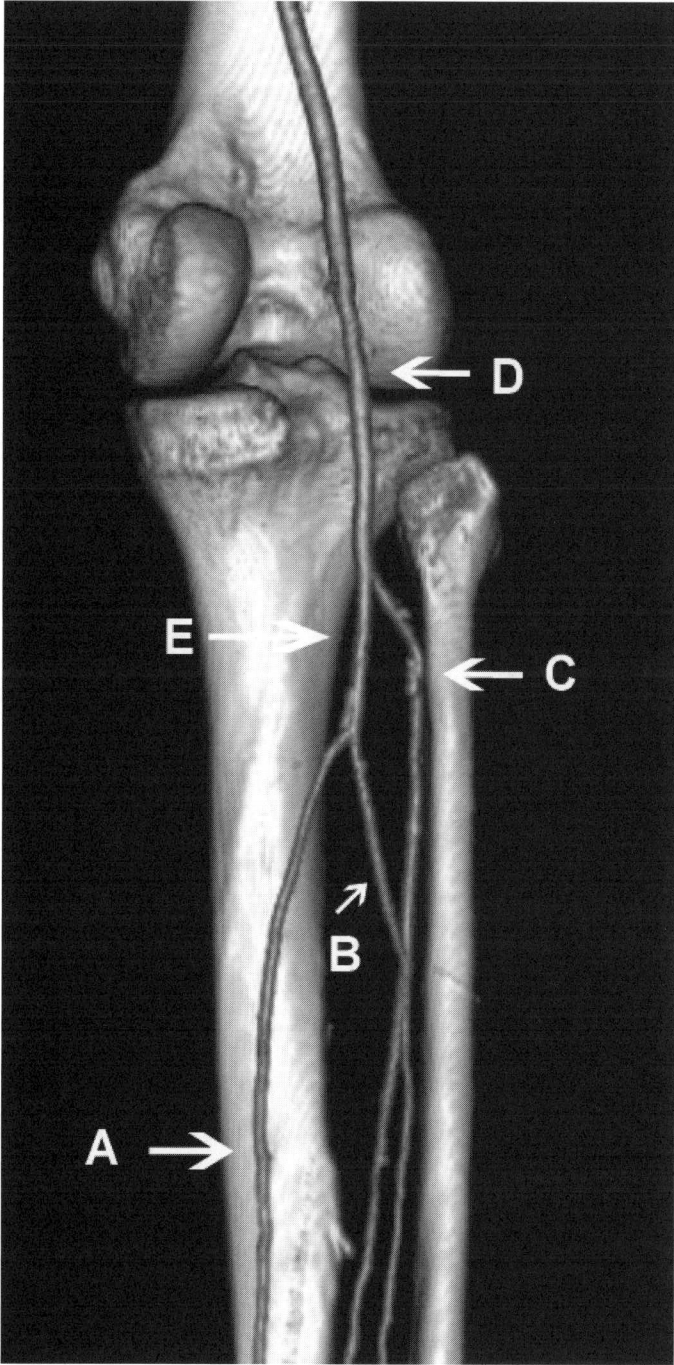

Figure 4-5. CTA of below the vessels. A. Posterior tibial artery. B. Peroneal artery. C. Anterior tibial artery. D. Popliteal artery. E. Tibioperoneal trunk

Advantages

Multi-detector CTA has high spatial resolution to depict vascular abnormality in fine details. Additional advantages of CTA include low cost (compared to MRA or catheter-based angiography), less physician dependency during imaging acquisition, faster scanning speed with minimal breath hold, short image acquisition time, and availability.

Disadvantages

Technical Factors
CTA requires the use of iodine-based contrast, which can cause contrast nephrotoxicity and/or allergic reaction. Other issues include radiation exposure and lengthy post-processing time.

Imaging Factors
Imaging limitations of CTA include the presence of dense calcifications and endoluminal stents, which may impair the quantification of the degrees of stenoses, similar to coronary CTA.

Indications

In addition to typical findings in a patient with PAD such as intermittent claudication, ischemic rest pain, ischemic ulceration, unexplained or recurrent atheroembolism, and suspected arterial aneurysms, CTA can also assess inflammatory and aneurysmal diseases, thromboembolic disease, vascular injury, dissection, spontaneous and iatrogenic, venous diseases, and congenital abnormalities in stasis and thrombosis.

Patient Preparation

Prior to CTA, patients are asked to discontinue metformin for at least 24 to 48 hours before the examination. In addition, patients are also asked to drink 1-2 quarts of water prior to the study to allow visualization of visceral walls. Barium contrast will interfere with the interpretation of the exam, and those who recently required oral barium are asked to wait for at least several days before CTA exam is performed. For patients with iodine or shellfish allergy, an alternative exam such as MRA or duplex may be recommended. However, pre-medication with steroids or histamine H_1 and H_2 blockers are often successful.

Assessment of Peripheral Arterial Bypass Grafts

Due to high spatial resolution and lack of motion artifacts, CTA is a promising modality in the evaluation of vascular graft patency. In a clinical study,

Willmann et al (15) investigated the technical feasibility of 4-slice MDCTA in the assessment of peripheral arterial bypass grafts and evaluated its accuracy and reliability in the detection of graft-related complications (graft stenosis, aneurysmal changes, and arteriovenous fistulae) in 65 consecutive patients with 85 peripheral arterial bypass grafts. When compared with duplex ultrasound and conventional DSA, sensitivity and specificity values of more than 95% were achieved with MDCT angiography for the diagnosis of arterial bypass graft-related complications.

Assessment of Arterial Injuries of Extremities

Direct-contrast material-enhanced angiography is the examination performed to assess arterial integrity in patients with extremity trauma. Angiography depicts injuries that require therapeutic intervention, such as occlusions, arteriovenous fistulas, and pseudoaneurysms. Generally considered safe, catheter-based angiography may be associated with complications that result from the procedure itself. In the setting of peripheral vascular trauma, MDCT angiography has been reported to be highly accurate in assessing complicated or partial occlusions, arteriovenous fistulae, intimal flaps, and psuedoaneursyms. Soto et al compared MDCT angiography with conventional angiography during a 19-month period in which 142 arterial segments in the proximal portions of the extremities of 139 patients were scanned with trauma to extremities. The sensitivity of MDCT angiography was 95%, and the specificity was 99% for presence of arterial injuries as compared to conventional angiography (16).

Invasive Angiography

Lower-extremity angiography represents the gold standard for diagnostic evaluation of lower-extremity PAD and generally is reserved for patients for whom an intervention is indicated. These indications include disabling intermittent claudication and critical limb ischemia.

Contemporary angiographic equipment allows for identifying the vascular structures by digital subtraction of structures not filling with radiocontrast medium, and the term "digital subtraction angiography" (DSA) and "invasive angiography" often are used interchangeably.

General Principles of Invasive Angiography

Invasive angiography is an X-ray—based procedure that utilizes contrast-mediated enhancement of the lumen of vascular structures. Invasive angiography provides clear diagnostic images using manually guided arterial catheter radio-contrast delivery. While the images provide clear delineation of arterial lumen contour, invasive angiography provides limited information regarding the vessel wall, plaque, or extravascular structures. It is useful to think of the resulting images as lumen-o-grams, while CTA and MRA additionally provide information on surrounding structures. Invasive angiography requires direct arterial access and therefore is accompanied by the associated risks, including vessel dissection, hematoma formation, ecchymoses, extra-vascular bleeding, and pseudoaneurysm formation. Visualization of both lower extremities is often accomplished by a single automated injection of contrast through a catheter positioned in the aorta superior to the renal arteries with subsequent visualization of the contrast run-off into the lower extremities. Hence, diagnostic angiography of the lower extremities is most commonly accomplished using an aortogram with runoff (Figure 4-6). In many circumstances, vessel segments below the inguinal ligament are inadequately opacified using aortogram with run-off alone; therefore, selective catheterization of the lower-extremity arteries using catheter manipulation is additionally performed and allows better definition of vessels. The decision to perform selective catheterization is made at the time of the procedure and always requires additional radiocontrast. As previously stated, the decision to refer for invasive angiography should be reached with the idea that surgical or endovascular intervention is indicated or if CTA/MRA is inconclusive.

Standard invasive angiography relies on the passage of iodine-based contrast material through vessels and depicts the X-ray shadow around the contrast. The resulting image is based on the differential passage of X-rays through tissues not containing contrast. Although the standard of care is to use iodine-based radio-contrast, some centers will selectively employ carbon dioxide (CO_2) contrast in patients with renal insufficiency in an effort to minimize contrast use. While CO_2 contrast is safe in experienced hands, image quality is not as clear, so CO_2 contrast is generally reserved for patients with severe renal insufficiency. Gadolinium contrast can also be used in select patients, but the cost and volume needed for routine studies is restrictive.

Arterial Access

Most commonly, access to the arterial system is achieved through the common femoral artery ventral to the femoral head. When visualization of the arteries in a single limb is desirable, the contralateral femoral artery is often chosen because it allows advancement of the catheter from the common iliac origin to the tibial vessels. Alternative arterial access approaches can be taken, such as via an upper-extremity artery, or an ipsilateral anterograde approach, which does not allow visualization of the iliac vessels.

Indications

The indications for invasive angiography of the lower extremities are presented in Table 4-1 and include lifestyle-limiting claudication, ischemic rest

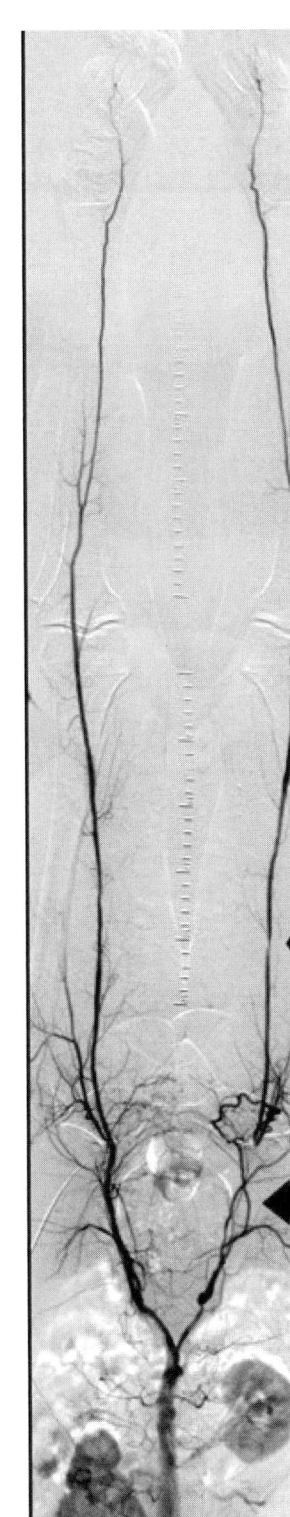

Figure 4-6. A composite invasive angiogram of the abdomen with lower extremity runoff provides a two dimensional view of the arterial lumen in a patient with multiple areas of lower extremity obstruction. Localized disease includes complete occlusion of the common femoral artery (upper arrow) and stenosis in the middle superficial femoral artery (lower arrow).

pain, and poorly healing ischemic ulceration. Invasive angiography is also performed when CTA or MRA provide equivocal results. In summary, contrast arteriography is performed when an intervention is planned, or if non-invasive imaging data is equivocal.

Contraindications

While there are no absolute contraindications, relative contraindications are well defined and are as follows.

Severe Renal Dysfunction

Patients with pre-existing renal dysfunction, dehydration, diabetes mellitus, congestive heart failure, and the elderly are the most susceptible to renal insult from iodinated contrast used in invasive angiography. Unfortunately, the majority of patients for whom angiography is indicated have at least one of these conditions, and adequate pre-hydration in these patients should be a major consideration.

Contrast Allergy

Screening for previous contrast allergy or shellfish allergy by questioning should always be performed prior to referral for invasive angiography. Patients for whom a positive or questionable allergy history exists should receive appropriate instruction regarding pre-medication, and the angiography lab should be notified for instruction on pre-medication. Both inpatient and outpatient pre-medication regimens have been devised and typically include histamine H_1 and H_2 blockers (diphenhydramine and ranitidine), as well as corticosteroids (prednisone or prednisolone).

Anticoagulant Agents

In general, antiplatelet agents such as aspirin, clopidogrel, or cilostazol do not need to be discontinued prior to angiography, although they do increase the risk of arterial access site hematoma or ecchymosis. In contrast, patients for whom invasive angiography is not urgent should have anticoagulants such as warfarin discontinued before arterial puncture. Patients taking warfarin for whom anticoagulation is considered essential can be admitted to the hospital 1-3 days prior to the procedure, with "bridging" with low-molecular-weight heparins. In such patients, heparin is discontinued 4-6 hours prior to the procedure and reinitiated once adequate hemostasis is achieved.

Uncontrolled Hypertension

Patients with uncontrolled hypertension (e.g. diastolic >100 mmHg) have an increased incidence of bleeding complications and should be controlled in the peri-procedural period.

Diabetes

Three distinct issues regarding diabetics should be considered prior to angiogram

1. Insulin usage: Each angiography laboratory should have a standard means of managing insulin and should be contacted for patient instruction. It is common place to ask outpatients coming to the interventional vascular laboratory to withhold insulin on the morning of the procedure. Inpatients can receive half-maintenance insulin with concomitant administration of dextrose-containing fluids.
2. Metformin usage: Because diabetics are at an increased risk of renal dysfunction after radio-contrast administration, and the risk of lactic acidosis is increased in patients taking Metformin, most patients are instructed to discontinue Metformin from the day of the procedure to at least 1 day after to ensure adequate return of renal function.
3. Hydration status: Dehydration and baseline renal dysfunction are common in diabetics and oral or IV hydration should be considered as a means to prevent contrast-mediated acute tubular necrosis.

Advantages

Invasive arteriography is the definitive procedure particularly to treat specific arterial stenoses and occlusions. A 2-dimensional representation of vessels allows for definitive vessel measurements and provides a clear roadmap for surgical or endovascular intervention. Identification of arterial inflow and runoff provide the interventionalist or surgeon a definitive assessment of the arterial anatomy relevant to revascularization. Specific flow characteristics are identified and are crucial to the clinical management of obstructive disease i.e. focal versus diffuse disease, embolic versus thrombotic, and atherosclerotic versus vasculitic.

Disadvantages

Despite the designation as "gold standard," invasive angiography has two distinct diagnostic drawbacks. First, standard invasive angiography provides a 2-dimensional or 'flat' depiction of the vessel lumen and poorly assesses the cross-sectional lumen area. Therefore, its ability to depict eccentric plaque is limited and may result in a false negative when true obstruction is present. To overcome this deficiency, some investigators have added intraluminal vascular ultrasound. Second, the diagnostic limitation of invasive angiography relates to its inability to visualize the vessel wall (intima, media, and adventia), where atherosclerosis has a significant impact. This

---

Table 4-2.   Complications of Invasive Angiography

- Pseudoaneurysm
- Retroperitoneal hemorrhage
- Hematoma
- Ecchymoses
- Pain
- Renal Failure
- Allergic reaction
- Bleeding
- Arterial embolization
- Access site obstruction
- Infection

---

disadvantage has particular importance when using invasive angiography in the presence of arterial aneurysms. Many aneurysms have extensive laminated plaque and thrombus that are not opacified by radiocontrast and alternative imaging; for example, duplex, CTA or MRA should be performed if aneurysm is suspected.

As the understanding of atherosclerosis increases, the focus on atherosclerotic plaque has intensified, and differentiation between stable and unstable plaque has received greater attention. In general, invasive angiography does not adequately allow differentiation of lipid-rich plaque from fibrotic scarred plaque. At this time however, current clinical practice is not significantly affected by atherosclerotic plaque appearance.

From a technical perspective, disadvantages of angiography relate to its invasiveness that requires direct arterial access and intra-arterial injection of iodinated radiocontrast. Furthermore, conscious sedation is commonly employed, and patients are required to have a means of transportation. The risks of invasive angiogram are summarized in Table 4-2. Commonly cited complications are pseudoaneurysm, retroperitoneal hemorrhage, hematoma, ecchymoses, pain, and bleeding. Additional risks include arterial embolization, access site obstruction, and infection.

Patient Preparation

Diagnostic lower-extremity angiography is often performed as a same-day procedure unless there is renal insufficiency or complications. Patients should be instructed to be NPO for 6-8 hours prior to the procedure except for medications. Patients should expect to receive some sedation and need to arrange means of transportation after the procedure. Post-procedure patients should expect to be fully supine for at least 4 hours to allow hemostasis at the arterial puncture site. Patients with diabetes, renal insufficiency, or those taking anticoagulants should notify the angiography lab and request specific instructions regarding medication management. Patients should have a creatinine and complete blood count documented generally within 1 month of the procedure.

Summary

High-resolution imaging of the lower-extremity arteries for PAD can be performed noninvasively using either MRA or CTA in most patients. Initial imaging of symptomatic patients with MRA or CTA can be performed to establish an anatomic diagnosis and a baseline anatomical map in anticipation of endovascular and/or surgical intervention.

REFERENCES
1. Criqui MH, Denenberg JO, Langer RD, Fronek A. The epidemiology of peripheral arterial disease: importance of identifying the population at risk. Vasc Med. 1997;2:221-6.
2. American Association for Vascular Surgery/Society for Vascular Surgery. ACC/AHA Guidelines for the Management of Patients with Peripheral Arterial Disease (lower extremity, renal, mesenteric, and abdominal aortic): a collaborative report from the American Associations for Vascular Surgery/Society for Vascular Surgery, Society for Cardiovascular Angiography and Interventions, Society for Vascular Medicine and Biology, Society of Interventional Radiology, and the ACC/AHA Task Force on Practice Guidelines (writing committee to develop guidelines for the management of patients with peripheral arterial disease)—summary of recommendations. J Vasc Interv Radiol. 2006;17:1383-97; quiz 1398.
3. Wedeen VJ, Meuli RA, Edelman RR, et al. Projective imaging of pulsatile flow with magnetic resonance. Science. 1985;230:946-8.
4. Leiner T. Magnetic resonance angiography of abdominal and lower extremity vasculature. Top Magn Reson Imaging. 2005;16:21-66.
5. Leiner T, Kessels AG, Nelemans PJ, et al. Peripheral arterial disease: comparison of color duplex US and contrast-enhanced MR angiography for diagnosis. Radiology. 2005;235:699-708.
6. Sadowski EA, Bennett LK, Chan MR, et al. Nephrogenic systemic fibrosis: risk factors and incidence estimation. Radiology. 2007;243:148-57.
7. Sam AD 2nd, Morasch MD, Collins J, et al. Safety of gadolinium contrast angiography in patients with chronic renal insufficiency. J Vasc Surg. 2003;38:313-8.
8. Yuan C, Kerwin WS, Ferguson MS, et al. Contrast-enhanced high resolution MRI for atherosclerotic carotid artery tissue characterization. J Magn Reson Imaging. 2002;15:62-7.
9. Rieker O, Düber C, Neufang A, et al. CT angiography versus intraarterial digital subtraction angiography for assessment of aortoiliac occlusive disease. AJR Am J Roentgenol. 1997;169:1133-8.
10. Rieker O, Düber C, Schmiedt W, et al. Prospective comparison of CT angiography of the legs with intraarterial digital subtraction angiography. AJR Am J Roentgenol. 1996;166:269-76.
11. Rubin GD, Schmidt AJ, Logan LJ, Sofilos MC. Multi-detector row CT angiography of lower extremity arterial inflow and runoff: initial experience. Radiology. 2001;221:146-58.
12. Rubin GD. Data explosion: the challenge of multidetector-row CT. Eur J Radiol. 2000;36:74-80.

13. **Martin ML, Tay KH, Flak B, et al.** Multidetector CT angiography of the aortoiliac system and lower extremities: a prospective comparison with digital subtraction angiography. AJR Am J Roentgenol. 2003;180:1085-91.
14. **Willmann JK, Wildermuth S, Pfammatter T, et al.** Aortoiliac and renal arteries: prospective intraindividual comparison of contrast-enhanced three-dimensional MR angiography and multi-detector row CT angiography. Radiology. 2003;226:798-811.
15. **Willmann JK, Mayer D, Banyai M, et al.** Evaluation of peripheral arterial bypass grafts with multi-detector row CT angiography: comparison with duplex US and digital subtraction angiography. Radiology. 2003;229:465-74.
16. **Soto JA, Múnera F, Cardoso N, et al.** Diagnostic performance of helical CT angiography in trauma to large arteries of the extremities. J Comput Assist Tomogr. 1999;23:188-96.

KEY REFERENCES

Fleischmann D, Hallett RL, Rubin GD. CT angiography of peripheral arterial disease. J Vasc Interv Radiol. 2006;17:3-26. *A technical manuscript serving as a comprehensive review for physicians performing CT angiography of the lower extremities.*

Kuo PH, et al. Gadolinium-based MR contrast agents and nephrogenic systemic fibrosis. Radiology. 2007;242:647-9. *A comprehensive editorial describing key issues relevant to use of gadolinium-containing contrast for patients with renal insufficiency from a medical foundation that maintains a registry for nephrogenic systemic fibrosis.*

Leiner T. Magnetic resonance angiography of abdominal and lower extremity vasculature. Top Magn Reson Imaging. 2005;16:21-66. *A comprehensive and detailed manuscript describing the development and the practical and theoretical aspects of MRA of the lower extremities.*

Ouwendijk R. et al. Imaging peripheral arterial disease: a randomized controlled trial comparing contrast-enhanced MR angiography and multi-detector row CT angiography. Radiology. 2005;236:1094-103. *A randomized trial of CTA vs. MRA for lower-extremity PAD with a focus on subsequent therapeutic outcomes and cost.*

Sun Z. Diagnostic accuracy of multislice CT angiography in peripheral arterial disease. J Vasc Interv Radiol. 2006;17:1915-21. *The publication is a concise and contemporary meta-analysis confirming the diagnostic utility of CT angiography with demonstration of improved accuracy with increased number of detectors.*

White C. Clinical practice. Intermittent claudication. N Engl J Med. 2007;356:1241-50. *A succinct case study with review that demonstrates the role of CTA, MRA, and angiography in patients with intermittent claudication.*

Chapter 5

Medical Treatment of Claudication and Critical Limb Ischemia

WENDY S. TZOU, MD
EMILE R. MOHLER III, MD

1. How do I manage peripheral arterial disease (PAD) risk factors?
2. What is the role of exercise therapy and how is it accomplished?
3. What pharmacotherapy will help improve claudication walking distance?
4. What are the appropriate treatment strategies for foot ulcers?
5. What are the strategies to prevent progression to critical limb ischemia?

Management of Peripheral Arterial Disease Risk Factors

PAD risk factors, the same as those for coronary heart disease (CHD), should be treated and managed aggressively once identified because they are common to the development of other manifestations of atherothrombotic disease, including myocardial infarction (MI) and stroke (Table 5-1). Major risk factors and associated management recommendations are detailed below.

Antiplatelet therapy, specifically in the form of aspirin and/or clopidogrel, is the foundation of pharmacologic management for PAD and atherosclerosis in general (1). These agents reduce risk of fatal myocardial infarction, ischemic stroke, and other vascular events by as much as 25%. Aspirin doses between 75 and 325 mg per day appear to represent the most effective therapy (2). Clopidogrel at 75 mg per day is also effective at reducing cardiovascular risk, with an almost 24% risk reduction reported over aspirin in the subset of PAD patients enrolled in the Clopidogrel Versus

---

Table 5-1.   Medical Treatment of Peripheral Arterial Disease

- Antiplatelet drug(s)
- Risk-factor modification
  - Smoking cessation
  - Strict glucose control if diabetic
  - Blood pressure control
  - Lipid modification (statins first line)
- Supervised exercise rehabilitation
- Cilostazol (Pletal)
- Foot care

Aspirin in Patients at Risk of Ischemic Events (CAPRIE) trial (3). The ACC/AHA guidelines and the TASC-2 guidelines both recommend antiplatelet therapy in all patients with PAD unless contraindicated.

No evidence currently exists that convincingly show that combination therapy among these patients is more effective than single-agent antiplatelet therapy in reducing cardiovascular disease (CVD) risk (1). The CHARISMA (Clopidogrel for High Atherothrombotic Risk and Ischemic Stabilization, Management and Avoidance) trial showed that the combination of the antiplatelet agents, clopidogrel and aspirin, did not demonstrate a statistically significant reduction in the risk of heart attack, stroke, or cardiovascular death compared to placebo and aspirin in a broad population of patients with either established atherothrombotic disease or multiple risk factors for atherothrombotic events. Analysis of the two enrollment subgroups, those with overt disease and those without, revealed different responses to clopidogrel and aspirin therapy. In patients with established atherothrombotic disease, the CHARISMA findings demonstrated that clopidogrel in addition to aspirin and other standard therapy reduced the relative risk of a recurrent heart attack (MI), stroke, or cardiovascular death by a statistically significant 12.5% (P=0.046) compared to patients receiving placebo and aspirin. These patients accounted for nearly 80% percent (n=12,153) of the total CHARISMA study population. Patients with multiple risk factors but no clearly established vascular disease did not benefit from the addition of clopidogrel to aspirin (20% relative risk increase, P=0.22). These patients represented approximately 20% (n=3,284) of the overall study population. In this patient subgroup, there was an excess in cardiovascular mortality as well as a non-statistically significant increase in bleeding observed in patients treated with clopidogrel and aspirin.

Ticlopidine has also been shown to decrease mortality and modestly improve intermittent claudication symptoms among PAD patients (4). However, its potential hematologic side effects (thrombocytopenia and leukopenia) require close monitoring for at least 3 months after initiating therapy.

Cigarette smoking has repeatedly been shown to be associated with PAD and is widely considered to be the most significant risk factor (5,6).

Multiple prospective studies have not only confirmed this 2- to 10-fold increased relative risk (RR), but have also demonstrated a dose-response effect (7). Smoking also accelerates the progression of claudication symptoms and increases the need for revascularization and amputation among those with known disease (8-10). Although no randomized, controlled trials have been conducted to confirm whether smoking cessation improves claudication symptoms, several studies have demonstrated improvements in walking distance and pain among those who discontinued tobacco use compared to those who continue to smoke (11,12). Additionally, a meta-analysis confirmed that smoking cessation improved bypass graft patency rates to those of never-smokers, even in those who stopped smoking after their lower-extremity graft surgery (10). Overall, there appears to be an improvement in the risk for vascular events with smoking cessation, particularly with respect to improved coronary event risk (13). Finally, PAD patients who continue to smoke have been shown to have a 40%-50% increased 10-year mortality from CHD or stroke (14,15).

Most-effective therapeutic strategies for smoking cessation include a multidisciplinary approach, incorporating education, structured counseling, and pharmacologic agents. The US Preventive Services Task Force (USPSTF) recommends viewing tobacco dependence as a chronic disease with recurrences and remissions, with relapse considered part of the disease instead of as failure in treatment (16). Furthermore, direct care-provider interventions, even in the form of brief counseling, appear to have significant effects on successful smoking cessation, particularly among motivated individuals and when followed up on multiple occasions (17). A standardized, clinical approach for facilitating smoking cessation has been outlined for identification and treatment based on patient characteristics (18). Assistance with non-pharmacologic therapies can be further provided by referral to dedicated smoking cessation programs or to various "quitlines," which provide free telephone counseling (19). Both are available in most states.

Multiple options for pharmacologic treatment are also available to augment counseling and behavioral modification. First-line agents that are approved by the US Food and Drug Administration (FDA) for tobacco dependence are nicotine replacement in the form of gum, patch, or spray and bupropion. If needed, both types can be combined for short-term use to aid in smoking cessation. All have approximately equal reported efficacy in smoking cessation (20,21), with quit rates varying from 50% to 100%. One newer agent, varenicline (Chantix), is a partial nicotinic acetylcholine receptor agonist. Varenicline is designed to partially activate this system while displacing nicotine at its sites of action in the brain. The typical treatment period is for 12 weeks. Although more patients remained smoke-free while taking the medication, the percentage of smokers who were smoke-free a year after quitting with varenicline ranged from 14% to 23% in clinical trials. One clinical trial indicated a higher quit rate with varenicline than buproprion; however, the importance of smoking cessation warrants multiple attempts with multiple drugs.

Second-line pharmacologic agents that are not FDA-approved for smoking cessation include clonidine and nortriptyline (18). These should only be considered in patients with contraindications for or lack of success with the first-line therapies. A promising investigational agent not yet available for clinical use is rimonobant, a type 1 cannabinoid receptor inhibitor that has shown efficacy in weight loss and smoking cessation (22).

Diabetes mellitus significantly increases the risk for PAD. The mechanism appears to be related to endothelial and vascular smooth muscle dysfunction that creates a prothrombotic milieu. PAD prevalence is 2-4 times higher among diabetic than non-diabetic patients (23-26). No study has definitively shown that strict glycemic control reduces macrovascular diabetic complications, including incident PAD or progression. However, a trend in reducing macrovascular events, specifically myocardial infarction, and a definite reduction in microvascular complications have been demonstrated, so strict glycemic control with a goal hemoglobin A1c of <7% is still strongly recommended (27). The Diabetes Control and Complications Trial/ Epidemiology of Diabetes Interventions and Complications (DCCT/EDIC) study research group data indicate an additional average 5.6 to 7.7 years in which patients are free from blindness, renal failure, and amputations and an increased life span by 5 years (27a). Additionally, proper foot care, hygiene, and immediate attention to any foot lesions or ulcerations should be incorporated as part of routine care (see below).

Medical treatment of dyslipidemia has been a mainstay of treatment in PAD (1,28), in part for its overall reduction in CVD risk. In the Heart Protection Study, for instance, 2701 PAD patients were enrolled among a total of 20,536 subjects at high risk for CVD events. Among those with PAD but no previous coronary heart disease, a small but significant (5.8%, $P<0.0001$) reduction in major vascular events was observed in those treated with simvastatin versus placebo, and an 18% reduction in CVD death was observed in those with an LDL cholesterol <116 mg/dL (29). Reductions in disease progression have also been shown. For example, treatment of 188 men with coronary artery disease and PAD with colestipol and niacin in the Cholesterol Lowering Atherosclerosis Study showed significant stabilization or even regression of angiographic femoral artery atherosclerosis (30), and the Regression Growth Evaluation Study (REGRESS) demonstrated that among 255 men with coronary artery disease carotid and femoral artery intima-media thickness, which predict CVD events, were reduced with pravastatin treatment compared to placebo (31).

Lipid lowering is not only beneficial in terms of reducing overall CVD risk, but symptoms may also be improved in the setting of treatment. For instance, a post-hoc subgroup analysis of the Scandinavian Simvastatin Survival Study (4S) showed that treatment with simvastatin was associated with a significant 38% risk reduction in development or worsening of intermittent claudication (32). Several clinical trials specifically designed to study lipid-lowering effects on claudication using statins have also been performed and demonstrated significant improvements in pain-free walking time after 3-12 months of treatment (33,34).

Therefore, lipid-lowering therapy, with a goal LDL cholesterol of <100 mg/dL generally, or <70 mg/dL among those at higher risk, should be initiated in all patients diagnosed with PAD (35). Higher-risk characteristics include those with multiple other risk factors, especially diabetes mellitus and/or other poorly controlled risk factors; presence of metabolic syndrome characteristics, including triglycerides >200 mg/dL or non-HDL cholesterol >130 mg/dL or HDL cholesterol <40 mg/dL in men or <50 mg/dL in women (28); or those with acute coronary syndromes. Statin therapy is recommended for all PAD patients without contraindications.

Hypertension is also a common finding in and risk factor for PAD (6,36). There have been few studies of blood pressure treatment enrolling only subjects with PAD. One study, The Heart Outcomes Prevention Evaluation (HOPE) Study, examined whether an angiotensin-converting enzyme (ACE) inhibitor (ramipril) could improve cardiovascular outcomes among high-risk patients with known cardiovascular disease and prospectively enrolled patients with PAD. The PAD subpopulation significantly benefited from ACE inhibition. Furthermore, multiple studies of blood pressure lowering that have included PAD patients indicate that strict blood pressure control, particularly among those with diabetes, effectively reduces CVD events (27,37). Therefore, antihypertensive therapy is advocated, with goal blood pressure <140/90 mmHg in non-diabetic patients, and <130/80 mmHg among those with diabetes. Among the latter group, ACE inhibition should be a mainstay of therapy. Beta-blockers across several randomized controlled trials have not been found to impair walking capacity compared to placebo and therefore are not contraindicated for blood pressure lowering among PAD subjects (38).

Role of Exercise Therapy and How It Is Accomplished

Exercise rehabilitation therapy has been shown to improve claudication symptoms. Walking distances before onset of pain have been reported to increase by as much as 179%, and distances walked before reaching maximal pain have been observed to increase by 122% (39). Among multiple randomized, controlled trials, exercise has not only been shown to significantly increase maximum walking time (mean difference 6.5 minutes), but benefits observed were greater than that seen with angioplasty at 6 months (mean difference 3.3 minutes) (40). Additionally, benefits in overall functional status, quality of life, and total caloric expenditures are associated with increased exercise. Patients should be referred to a claudication exercise rehabilitation program. Supervised walking sessions of at least 45-60 minutes each, occurring >3 times/week, achieving near-maximal claudication pain, and performed consistently for at least 6 months are recommended for symptomatic PAD patients (1,39). The supervising exercise physiologist, physical therapist, or nurse monitors the individual patient's claudication threshold and other cardiovascular limitations to adjust workload. Interim development of arrhythmias, angina, or continued inability of the patient to progress to an adequate level of exercise may prompt further physician review. Patients who show improvement usually do so within about 2 months of consistent therapy; stopping therapy decreases potential gains. Promise has additionally been demonstrated among unsupervised exercise, which is an alternative when transportation, cost, or scheduling conflicts prevent enrollment into a supervised program. A recent study of 417 PAD patients reported that those reporting walking >3 times per week or >90 minutes per week had a significantly lower annual decline in 6-minute walking distance than those reporting less or no weekly exercise (41).

Pharmacotherapy for Improved Claudication Walking Distance

Cilostazol, a type 3 phosphodiesterase inhibitor, improves maximal walking distance by as much as 40%-60% over a 3-6 month treatment period (1). Benefits in functional status and quality of life, as well as slight improvement in ABI may be achieved with this drug (42,43). Treatment with 100 mg twice daily is currently recommended for those with lifestyle-limiting claudication, and improvements in symptoms may be observed after as little as 4 weeks of treatment (42,44). However, the FDA warns that this agent should not be used in those with heart failure. Although not tested in patients with history of heart failure, detrimental effects have been observed in such patients treated long-term with other drugs of this class. The most common side effects from cilostazol are headache, palpitations, and diarrhea.

Pentoxifylline, a methylxanthine derivative taken at 400 mg three times per day, may be a second-line agent to cilostazol to consider because it has been shown to marginally improve walking distances (34). However, the observed and expected improvements are modest at best, and, as with cilostazol, symptomatic improvement may not occur until after at least 4 weeks of treatment.

Appropriate Treatment Strategies for Foot Ulcers

The prevalence of concurrent PAD, foot ulcers, and diabetes mellitus has not been specifically determined, although they are known to be highly associated. Data from the 1999-2000 National Health and Examination Survey (NHANES) indicate that the prevalence of PAD among diabetic patients is twice that of the overall population, and the prevalence of ulcers is nearly three times as high (25). Care of the PAD patient with a diabetic foot ulcer must address tight glycemic control, weight loss and exercise as permitted, and other strategies previously discussed that are targeted to minimize macrovascular complications. Additionally, the following general foot care techniques can be utilized to help promote healing and prevent progression.

Relieving the pressure load on ulcers, commonly known as mechanical offloading, is a fundamental component of treatment (45). Ulcers formed on the plantar surface of the foot are more common among diabetic neuropathic feet and may be treated successfully with specially fitted orthotic devices such as total contact casts or special insoles or orthotics with load-isolation regions, all of which distribute body weight more evenly and off of the affected region (45). Ischemic or neuroischemic ulcers more commonly present on non-plantar surfaces, especially on the foot margins. Common locations are on the medial first metatarsophalangeal joint and over the lateral fifth metatarsophalangeal joint (46). These are similarly treated using by offloading, using footwear such as half-shoes or molded shoes with relief cut-outs overlying the lesion (45). Early identification and application of these principles to pre- or early ulcers may prevent development into deeper ulcers and subsequent complications. Pre-ulcers often present as areas of focal erythema due to friction from footwear. Without intervention, they may progress to superficial blisters and then to shallow ulcers with a yellow granulomatous base (46).

Once ulcers have formed, sharp wound debridement using a scalpel is indicated in order to remove sloughing skin, callous, and necrotic tissue, as their presence delays healing and promotes further ulceration, tissue necrosis, and infection (46). In the severely ischemic foot (ankle-brachial index <0.5), debridement should proceed cautiously so as not to remove viable tissue as well. Maggots have been used to debride severely neuroischaemic feet and may accelerate healing and mitigate infection (45,46). Newer investigational treatments include application of bone-marrow-derived stem cells (See chapter 8), recombinant human platelet-derived growth factor, negative pressure dressings, or bioengineered skin grafts (45). Hyperbaric oxygen may decrease risk for major amputation but does not appear to affect wound healing any more favorably than other novel modalities (47). In debriding wounds, examining for deeper ulcer or sinus tract extension using a blunt-tip probe is important to unmask potential deep wound infections, including osteomyelitis. The latter would then prompt further antimicrobial treatment and work-up for possible surgical debridement or amputation.

Infected foot ulcers, defined by the presence of purulent drainage with or without multiple signs of inflammation, such as erythema, warmth, tenderness, edema, or foul odor (45) should be promptly debrided and drained as needed. Tissue cultures or sterile fluid aspirates should be collected when possible to help tailor antimicrobial therapy because colonization by skin organisms render simple wound swabs less useful in terms of diagnosis (48). The most significant pathogenic organisms include gram-positive cocci, especially *Staphylococcus aureus*, coagulase-negative Staphylococci, and beta-hemolytic Streptococci. Mixed infections may also include obligate anaerobes. Oral antibiotic therapy should be initiated for mild-to-moderate infections; severe infections require prompt hospitalization, debridement, and parenteral antibiotics. Therapy should be initiated empirically and then tailored based on available culture results, clinical response, or suspicion for resistant organisms, particularly methicillin-resistant *Staphylococcus aureus* (45).

Strategies to Prevent Progression to Critical Limb Ischemia

The key step required to prevent progression of PAD is identification. Despite recent estimates that nearly 8 million Americans are afflicted (49), the disease remains clinically under-recognized and thus undertreated (50). Once PAD has been identified, aggressive risk factor management and preventative strategies using the guidelines described above are the key to preventing progression to critical limb ischemia.

REFERENCES

1. Hirsch AT, Haskal ZJ, Hertzer NR. ACC/AHA guidelines for the management of patients with peripheral arterial disease (lower extremity, renal, mesenteric, and abdominal aortic): executive summary: a report of the American College of Cardiology/American Heart Association Task Force on Practice Guidelines (Writing Committee to Develop Guidelines for the Management of Patients With Peripheral Arterial Disease [Lower Extremity, Renal, Mesenteric, and Abdominal Aortic]). J Am Coll Cardiol. 2006.

2. Antithrombotic Trialists' Collaboration. Collaborative meta-analysis of randomised trials of antiplatelet therapy for prevention of death, myocardial infarction, and stroke in high risk patients. BMJ. 2002;324:71-86.

3. CAPRIE Steering Committee. A randomised, blinded, trial of clopidogrel versus aspirin in patients at risk of ischaemic events (CAPRIE). Lancet. 1996;348:1329-39.

4. Girolami B, Bernardi E, Prins MH, et al. Antithrombotic drugs in the primary medical management of intermittent claudication: a meta-analysis. Thromb Haemost. 1999;81:715-22.

5. McDermott MM, Liu K, Criqui MH, et al. Ankle-brachial index and subclinical cardiac and carotid disease: the multi-ethnic study of atherosclerosis. Am J E. 2005;162:33-41.

6. Selvin E, Erlinger TP. Prevalence of and risk factors for peripheral arterial disease in the United States: results from the National Health and Nutrition Examination Survey, 1999-2000. Circulation. 2004;110:738-43.

7. Celermajer DS, Adams MR, Clarkson P, et al. Passive exposure to tobacco smoke impairs endothelium-dependent arterial dilatation in healthy young adults, which likely predisposes to atherogenesis. N Engl J Med. 1996;334:150-4.

8. Gardner AW. The effect of cigarette smoking on exercise capacity in patients with intermittent claudication. Vasc Med. 1996;1:181-6.

9. Katzel LI, Sorkin JD, Powell CC, Gardner AW. Comorbidities and exercise capacity in older

patients with intermittent claudication. Vasc Med. 2001;6:157-62.

10. **Willigendael EM, Teijink JA, Bartelink ML, et al.** Smoking and the patency of lower extremity bypass grafts: a meta-analysis. J Vasc Surg. 2005;42:67-74.

11. **Jonason T, Bergstrom R.** Cessation of smoking in patients with intermittent claudication. Effects on the risk of peripheral vascular complications, myocardial infarction and mortality. Acta Med Scand. 1987;221:253-60.

12. **Quick CR, Cotton LT.** The measured effect of stopping smoking on intermittent claudication. Br J Surg. 1982;69(Suppl):S24-S26.

13. **Hiatt WR.** Medical treatment of peripheral arterial disease and claudication. N Engl J Med. 2001;344:1608-21.

14. **Reunanen A, Takkunen H, Aromaa A.** Prevalence of intermittent claudication and its effect on mortality. Acta Med Scand. 1982;211:249-56.

15. **Faulkner KW, House AK, Castleden WM.** The effect of cessation of smoking on the accumulative survival rates of patients with symptomatic peripheral vascular disease. Med J Aust. 1983;1:217-19.

16. **Fiore MC, Bailey WC, Cohen SJ.** Treating tobacco use and dependence. Clinical Practice Guideline. Rockville, MD: US Department of Health and Human Services; 2000.

17. **Pinto BM, Rabin C, Farrell N.** Lifestyle and coronary heart disease prevention. Prim Care. 2005;32:947-61.

18. http://www surgeongeneral gov/tobacco/tobaqrg pdf, accessed 6/27/06. 2007.

19. **Zhu SH, Anderson CM, Tedeschi GJ, et al.** Evidence of real-world effectiveness of a telephone quitline for smokers. N Engl J Med. 2003;347:1087-93.

20. **Jorenby DE, Leischow SJ, Nides MA, et al.** A controlled trial of sustained-release bupropion, a nicotine patch, or both for smoking cessation. N Engl J Med. 1999;340:685-91.

21. **Silagy C, Lancaster T, Stead L, et al.** Nicotine replacement therapy for smoking cessation. Cochrane Database Syst Rev. 2004;3:CD000146.

22. **Gelfand EV, Cannon CP.** Rimonabant: a cannabinoid receptor type 1 blocker for management of multiple cardiometabolic risk factors. J Am Coll Cardiol. 2006;47: 1919-26.

23. **Beckman JA, Creager MA, Libby P.** Diabetes and atherosclerosis: epidemiology, pathophysiology, and management. JAMA. 2002;287:2570-2581.

24. **Eason SL, Petersen NJ, Suarez-Almazor M, et al.** Diabetes mellitus, smoking, and the risk for asymptomatic peripheral arterial disease: whom should we screen? J Am Board Fam Pract. 2005;18:355-61.

25. **Gregg EW, Sorlie P, Paulose-Ram R, et al.** Prevalence of lower-extremity disease in the US adult population =40 years of age with and without diabetes: 1999-2000 national health and nutrition examination survey. Diabetes Care. 2004;27:1591-7.

26. **Ness J, Aronow WS, Newkirk E, McDaniel D.** Prevalence of symptomatic peripheral arterial disease, modifiable risk factors, and appropriate use of drugs in the treatment of peripheral arterial disease in older persons seen in a university general medicine clinic. J Gerontol A Biol Sci Med Sci. 2005;60:255-7.

27. **UK Prospective Diabetes Study Group.** Intensive blood-glucose control with sulphonylureas or insulin compared with conventional treatment and risk of complications in patients with type 2 diabetes (UKPDS 33). Br Med J. 1998;352:837-53.

27a. **Narayan KM.** Cost-effectiveness of intensive insulin therapy in the Diabetes Control and Complications Trial. JAMA. 1997 Feb 5;277:374-5.

28. **Executive Summary of The Third Report of The National Cholesterol Education Program (NCEP) Expert Panel on Detection, Evaluation, and Treatment of High Blood Cholesterol in Adults (Adult Treatment Panel III).** JAMA. 2001;285:2486-97.

29. **MRC/BHF Heart Protection Study of cholesterol lowering with simvastatin in 20,536 high-risk individuals: a randomised placebo-controlled trial.** Lancet. 2002;360:7-22.

30. **Blankenhorn DH, Azen SP, Crawford DW, et al.** Effects of colestipol-niacin therapy on human femoral atherosclerosis. Circulation. 1991;83:438-47.

31. de GE, Jukema JW, Montauban van Swijndregt AD, et al. B-mode ultrasound assessment of pravastatin treatment effect on carotid and femoral artery walls and its correlations with coronary arteriographic findings: a report of the Regression Growth Evaluation Statin Study (REGRESS). J Am Coll Cardiol. 1998;31:1561-7.

32. Pedersen TR, Kjekshus J, Pyorala K, et al. Effect of simvastatin on ischemic signs and symptoms in the Scandinavian simvastatin survival study (4S). Am J Cardiol. 1998; 81:333-5.

33. Aronow WS, Nayak D, Woodworth S, Ahn C. Effect of simvastatin versus placebo on treadmill exercise time until the onset of intermittent claudication in older patients with peripheral arterial disease at six months and at one year after treatment. Am J Cardiol. 2003;92:711-12.

34. Mohler ER III. Peripheral arterial disease: identification and implications. Arch Intern Med. 2003;163:2306-14.

35. Grundy SM, Cleeman JI, Merz CN, et al. Implications of recent clinical trials for the National Cholesterol Education Program Adult Treatment Panel III guidelines. Arterioscler Thromb Vasc Biol. 2004;24:14961.

36. Mohler ER, Hiatt WR, Creager MA. Cholesterol reduction with atorvastatin improves walking distance in patients with peripheral vascular disease. Circulation. 2002;106.

37. Mehler PS, Coll JR, Estacio R, et al. Intensive blood pressure control reduces the risk of cardiovascular events in patients with peripheral arterial disease and type 2 diabetes. Circulation. 2003;107:753-6.

38. Radack K, Deck C. Beta-adrenergic blocker therapy does not worsen intermittent claudication in subjects with peripheral arterial disease. A meta-analysis of randomized controlled trials [see comments]. Arch Intern Med. 1991;151:1769-76.

39. Gardner AW, Poehlman ET. Exercise rehabilitation programs for the treatment of claudication pain. A meta-analysis. JAMA. 1995;274:975-80.

40. Leng GC, Fowler B, Ernst E. Exercise for intermittent claudication. Cochrane Database Syst Rev. 2000;2:CD000990.

41. McDermott MM, Liu K, Ferrucci L, et al. Physical performance in peripheral arterial disease: a slower rate of decline in patients who walk more. Ann Intern Med. 2006;144: 10-20.

42. Mohler ER III, Beebe HG, Salles-Cuhna S, et al. Effects of cilostazol on resting ankle pressures and exercise-induced ischemia in patients with intermittent claudication. Vasc Med. 2001;6:151-6.

43. Regensteiner JG, Ware JE Jr., McCarthy WJ, et al. Effect of cilostazol on treadmill walking, community-based walking ability, and health-related quality of life in patients with intermittent claudication due to peripheral arterial disease: meta-analysis of six randomized controlled trials. J Am Geriatr Soc. 2002;50:1939-46.

44. Reilly MP, Mohler ER III. Cilostazol: treatment of intermittent claudication. Ann Pharmacother. 2001;35:48-56.

45. Cavanagh PR, Lipsky BA, Bradury AW, Botek G. Treatment for diabetic foot ulcers. Lancet. 2005;366:1725-35.

46. Edmonds M, Foster AV. Diabetic foot ulcers. Br Med J. 2006;332:407-10.

47. Roeckl-Wiedmann I, et al. Systematic review of hyperbaric oxygen in the management of chronic wounds. Br J Surg. 2005;92:24-32.

48. Bowler PG, et al. Wound microbiology and associated approaches to wound management. Clin Microbiol Rev. 2001;14:244-69.

49. Allison MA, Criqui MH, Ho E, Denenberg JO. The estimated ethnic-specific prevalence of peripheral arterial disease in the United States, 2000. Circulation. 2004;110(Suppl III):III-817. 2004.

50. Hirsch AT, Criqui MH, Treat-Jacobson D, Peripheral arterial disease detection, awareness, and treatment in primary care. JAMA. 2001;286:1317-24.

KEY REFERENCES

Hirsch AT, Haskal ZJ, Hertzer NR. ACC/AHA guidelines for the management of patients with peripheral arterial disease (lower extremity, renal, mesenteric, and abdominal aortic): executive summary: a report of the American College of Cardiology/American Heart Association Task Force on Practice Guidelines (Writing Committee to Develop Guidelines for the Management of Patients With Peripheral Arterial Disease [Lower Extremity, Renal, Mesenteric, and Abdominal Aortic]). J Am Coll Cardiol. 2006. *Comprehensive guidelines for diagnosis and treatment of peripheral arterial disease.*

Antithrombotic Trialists' Collaboration. Collaborative meta-analysis of randomised trials of antiplatelet therapy for prevention of death, myocardial infarction, and stroke in high risk patients. Br Med J. 2002;324:71-86. *A meta-analysis that supports 325 mg of aspirin per day will reduce cardiovascular events in patients with claudication by approximately 25%.*

CAPRIE Steering Committee. A randomised, blinded, trial of clopidogrel versus aspirin in patients at risk of ischaemic events (CAPRIE). Lancet. 1996;348:1329-39. *A randomized study comparing apsirin 325 mg per day to clopidogrel 75 mg per day in patients with a history of symptomatic atherosclerotic disease including claudication. At 36 months the combined endpoint of myocardial infarction, cerebrovascular accident and death was reduced by approximately 9% in the clopidogrel treatment group compared to apspirin treatment group.*

Norgren L, Hiatt WR, Dormandy JA, et al. Inter-Society Consensus for the Management of Peripheral Arterial Disease (TASC II). J Vasc Surg. 2007;45:S5-S67. *International guidelines for diagnosing and treating peripheral arterial disease.*

Jonason T, Bergstrom R. Cessation of smoking in patients with intermittent claudication. Effects on the risk of peripheral vascular complications, myocardial infarction and mortality. Acta Med Scand. 1987;221:253-60. *Study that indicates smoking cessation results in improved mortality in patients with claudication.*

Mohler ER III. Therapy insight: peripheral arterial disease and diabetes: from pathogenesis to treatment guidelines. Nat Clin Pract Cardiovasc Med. 2007;4:151-62. *Review article that describes the pathophysiology of diabetic vasculopathy and treatment of this condition.*

MRC/BHF Heart Protection Study of cholesterol lowering with simvastatin in 20,536 high-risk individuals: a randomised placebo-controlled trial. Lancet. 2002;360:7-22. *First prospective study showing that statin treatment reduces cardiovascular risk in patients with PAD.*

Mohler ER III. Peripheral arterial disease: identification and implications. Arch Intern Med. 2003;163:2306-14.

Gardner AW, Poehlman ET. Exercise rehabilitation programs for the treatment of claudication pain. A meta-analysis. JAMA. 1995;274:975-80. *A meta-analysis showing that exercise rehabilitation improves pain-free walking distance in patients with claudication.*

Reilly MP, Mohler ER III. Cilostazol: treatment of intermittent claudication. Ann Pharmacother. 2001;35:48-56. *Review article describing the mechanism of action, clinical study data and potential side effects of cilostazol.*

Cavanagh PR, Lipsky BA, Bradury AW, Botek G. Treatment for diabetic foot ulcers. Lancet. 2005;366:1725-35. *An article describing the treatment of diabetic foot ulcers.*

Hirsch AT, Criqui MH, Treat-Jacobson D, et al. Peripheral arterial disease detection, awareness, and treatment in primary care. JAMA. 2001;286:1317-24. *A large prospective study evaluating the prevalence of PAD and PAD risk factors.*

Chapter 6

Endovascular Treatment of Intermittent Claudication and Critical Limb Ischemia

SALMAN ARAIN, MD
CHRISTOPHER J. WHITE, MD

1. **When should I consider endovascular therapy for aortoiliac?**
2. **When should I consider endovascular therapy for femoral-popliteal?**
3. **When should I consider endovascular therapy for tibioperoneal?**
4. **What are the complications and risks of endovascular therapy?**
5. **What are the adjuvent medical therapies for endovascular therapy?**

The mainstay of therapy for peripheral arterial disease (PAD) consists of atherosclerotic risk-factor modification in conjunction with antiplatelet therapy and a supervised exercise program. Additional pharmacologic therapy is warranted for symptomatic relief in stable patients who do not respond adequately to lifestyle modification and exercise therapy. Endovascular or surgical revascularization is reserved for symptomatic patients with critical limb ischemia and claudicators whose job performance or lifestyle is compromised by ischemic symptoms, and who fail medical therapy (1,2).

Distinguishing patients with claudication from the more malignant critical limb ischemia has a significant impact on revascularization strategies. Patients with claudication have a low (= 2%) risk of limb loss, whereas patients with critical limb ischemia, rest pain, non-healing lesions or gangrene) are at much higher risk of limb loss (Table 6-1). Treatment of claudication is directed towards symptom relief and restoration of limb function, whereas treatment of critical limb ischemia is directed towards

Table 6-1.   Factors That Predispose to Limb Loss in Patients Presenting with Critical Limb Ischemia (1)

Factors that reduce blood flow to the microvascular bed:
- Diabetes
- Severe renal failure
- Severely decreased cardiac output (severe heart failure or shock)
- Vasospastic diseases or concomitant conditions (e.g., Raynaud's phenomenon, prolonged cold exposure)
- Smoking and tobacco use

Factors that increase demand for blood flow to the microvascular bed:
- Infection (e.g., cellulitis, osteomyelitis)

Skin breakdown or traumatic injury

limb salvage, i.e. avoiding amputation. Both categories of patients are at very high risk of cardiovascular events from atherosclerosis (stroke, death, and myocardial infarction), making risk factor and lifestyle modification a crucial element of their treatment strategy (1-4).

Overview of Endovascular Therapy

Patients with symptomatic claudication, selected for elective percutaneous transluminal angioplasty (PTA), should have limitation of their lifestyle and/or be unable to work, having failed to respond to conservative therapy (medication and supervised exercise), with an anatomically suitable lesion for intervention (1). For critical limb ischemia, urgent revascularization with either surgery or endovascular therapy is indicated. In patients with threatened limb loss, transient restoration of blood flow often allows adequate perfusion to heal an ischemic ulcer. If there is no recurrent injury, the healed ulcer will not recur even if renarrowing (restenosis) occurs. Another indication for endovascular therapy is to repair or correct vascular access site complications following invasive procedures (Figure 6-1). In such patients, diagnostic angiography from the contralateral femoral artery or from the upper extremity will often confirm a "culprit" lesion, including a bleeding site, pseudoaneurysm, arteriovenous fistula, or thrombosis. Endovascular therapy is typically not indicated in asymptomatic patients. However, asymptomatic lesions may become candidates for intervention if the procedure facilitates intra-aortic counterpulsation balloon placement, or to allow access for coronary and/or carotid artery interventions.

There are no absolute contraindications to endovascular intervention. Relative contra-indications include lesions likely to generate atheroemboli, lesions that are heavily calcified and may be difficult to dilate, and instances in which the risks of the procedure, such as worsening of renal function, may outweigh the potential benefits.

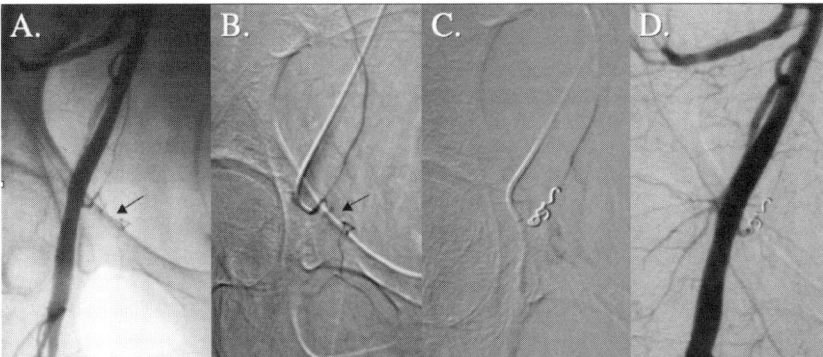

Figure 6-1. A patient with post-procedure hypotension and right groin fullness and tenderness after right femoral artery arterial access. A. Left femoral arterial access to contralateral femoral artery demonstrating extravasation from a small sidebranch (arrow). B. Seletive engagement of sidebranch with 6 Fr. Internal mammary catheter to localize extravasation (arrow). C. Placement of coils via the mammary catheter. D. Final angiogram demonstrating occlusion of the sidebranch to stop bleeding.

Patient Selection

In addition to the functional criteria listed above, patient selection for endovascular therapy depends upon several anatomic and clinical characteristics (Table 6-2). Anatomic criteria include the ability to gain vascular access, a reasonable likelihood of crossing the lesion with a guidewire, and the expectation that a catheter can be advanced to the lesion. The ability to pass a guidewire across the lesion is the rate-limiting step in all endovascular interventions, and a favorable procedural result is more likely for a stenosis than for an occlusion. Other anatomic criteria that affect outcomes following revascularization include increasing lesion length, the presence of multiple lesions, chronic total occlusions, and the coexistence of 'inflow' and 'outflow' disease. Multilevel disease is typically seen in patients presenting with critical limb ischemia. Patency rates following

Table 6-2.   Anatomic and Clinical Characteristics That Affect the Results of PTA

Favorable	*Unfavorable*
• Stenotic lesion	• Occlusion
• Non-calcified	• Long lesions ($\geq$5 cm)
• Discrete ($\leq$3 cm)	• Aorto-iliac aneurysm
• Patent run-off vessels ($\geq$2)	• Atheroembolic diseass
• Non-diabetic patients	• Extensive bilateral aorto-iliac disease

PTA = percutaneous transluminal angioplasty.

angioplasty are highest for stenoses with the iliac arteries, and decrease with distal disease sites. Clinical features that affect outcomes include the presence of diabetes, renal insufficiency, and smoking. Patients who present with critical limb ischemia have worse outcomes than those with less severe symptoms.

Technology Issues

The availability of endovascular stents has significantly extended the anatomic subset of patients that may be considered candidates for percutaneous revascularization, particularly longer lesions and occlusions (Table 6-3). Several stent technologies have been introduced in an effort to pro-

Table 6-3.   Overview of Technology Used in Lower-Extremity Interventions

Technology	Advantages	Disadvantages
PTA	• Low cost • Easy availability	• Variable patency rates, often lower in complex, longer, or calcified lesions
Balloon-expandable stents	• Eliminate technical failure from PTA-induced dissections or suboptimal vessel expansion • Can be positioned more precisely than self-expanding stents, which is an advantage in treating ostial lesions	• Stent 'failure' from thrombosis and restenosis • Risk of external compression outside of axial skeleton
Self-expanding Stents	• Have greater flexibility and 'shape memory' to resist external deformation • Newer generations have shown improved patency rates compared to angioplasty alone in SFA	• Substantial rate of stent fracture (up to 24%) in some vessels (e.g., the superficial femoral artery), which promotes restenosis and predisposes to late stent failure
Drug-eluting stents	• Theoretical reduction in intimal hyperplasia, and improved late patency	• High cost • Have not shown clinical superiority over bare metal stents • No evidence to show that they cause less restenosis than other stent types
Bioabsorbable stents	• Stents slowly get 'absorbed,' theoretically restoring vessel compliance and preventing chronic inflammation at the site of implantation	• Not enough clinical data to support their routine use • Higher rates of thrombosis and emboli
Stent grafts	• Slight improvement in patency over bare stents	

PTA = percutaneous transluminal angioplasty.

long the durability of percutaneous interventions by minimizing late stent failure from restenosis. Stent types currently being investigated include self-expanding stents, balloon-expandable stents, covered stents (i.e., stent grafts), drug-eluting stents, and bioabsorbable stents.

Endovascular Therapy for Aorto-Iliac Disease

Ideal patient and lesion subsets for iliac PTA have been proposed (Table 6-2) (5). The procedural success rate for balloon angioplasty of these "optimal" aorto-iliac lesions is expected to be >90%, with a 5-year patency rate of 54% to 78% (6-8). The procedural success (78% to 98%) and long-term patency (48% to 85%) rates are lower for occlusions than for stenoses (9,10). These results compare favorably with surgical results in patients following aortoiliac and aortofemoral bypass revascularization, which have a 74% to 95% 5-year patency (Table 6-4) (11,12). A randomized comparison of PTA versus surgery for 157 iliac lesions reported no difference in the 3-year cumulative rate for study-related deaths, amputations, and revascularization failure between surgery (Figure 6-2) (13). Randomized controlled trials comparing surgery to angioplasty demonstrate no difference at 1 to 3 years for the hemodynamic effect (Figure 6-3) (13,14). Therefore, the current recommendation, based upon these clinical trials, is to attempt percutaneous therapy first if the patient is a candidate for either procedure.

The advent of stents has improved the results of balloon angioplasty in aorto-iliac vessels (15-17). There has been debate about whether stent architecture, stent design, or the composition, i.e. nitinol versus stainless steel, has any effect on restenosis rates. The CRISP trial failed to show any difference in outcomes between nitinol (Smart, Cordis, Miami Lakes, FL) and stainless steel (Wallstent, Boston Scientific Corp., Watertown, MA) iliac artery stents at 1 year (Figure 6-4) (18). The result of primary iliac stent placement (without regard to the predilation balloon result) of balloon-expandable stents has been reported in a multicenter trial in 486 patients followed for up to 4 years (mean 13.3 ± 11 months) (19). Using a life-table analysis, clinical benefit was present in 91% of the patients at 1 year, 84%

Table 6-4.   Patency after Iliac PTA by Clinical and Lesion Variables (11)

	One-Year Patency (%)	Three-Year Patency (%)	Five-Year Patency (%)
Stenosis/claudication/good run-off	81	70	63
Stenosis/critical limb/poor run-off	65	48	38
Occlusion/claudication/good run-off	61	43	33
Occlusion/critical limb/poor run-off	56	17	10

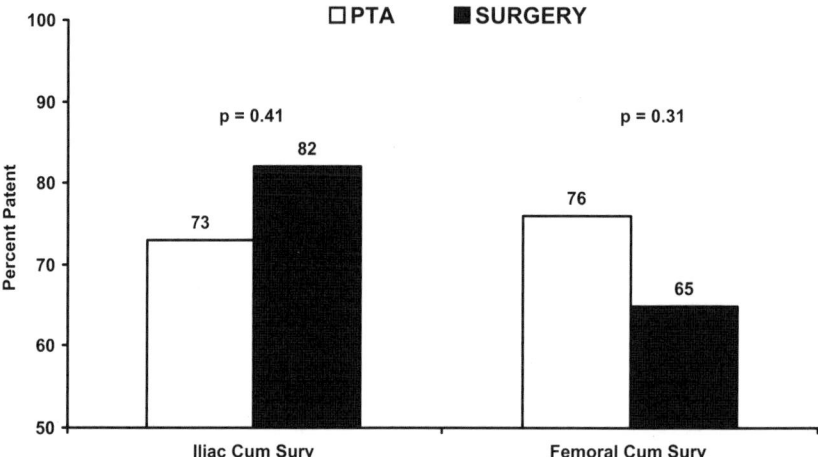

Figure 6-2.   Data from a randomized controlled trial showing no difference between surgery or PTA for amputation-free survival over three years. Wilson, S.E., G.L. Wolf, and A.P. Cross, Percutaneous transluminal angioplasty versus operation for peripheral arteriosclerosis. Report of a prospective randomized trial in a selected group of patients. J Vasc Surg, 1989. 9(1): p. 1-9.

at 2 years, and 69% at 43 months of follow-up. The angiographic patency rate of the iliac stents was 92%.

Stent placement following a suboptimal angioplasty result (provisional stent placement) has been reported in 184 iliac lesions after failed or suboptimal balloon angioplasty outcomes (20). A 91% procedural success rate and a 6-month patency rate of 99% was achieved for iliac lesions. Long-term follow-up demonstrated a 4-year primary patency rate of 86% and a secondary patency rate of 95% for iliac arteries. Excellent results for provisional

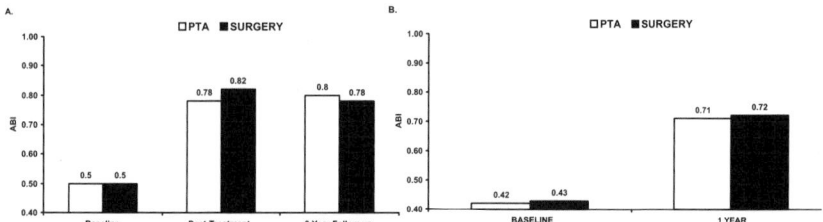

Figure 6-3.   Randomized controlled trials, Panel A of Wilson et al and Panel B of Holm et al comparing surgery to PTA with no difference in hemodynamic results (ABI = ankle-brachial index). Wilson, S.E., G.L. Wolf, and A.P. Cross, Percutaneous transluminal angioplasty versus operation for peripheral arteriosclerosis. Report of a prospective randomized trial in a selected group of patients. J Vasc Surg, 1989. 9(1): p. 1-9 and Holm, J., et al., Chronic lower limb ischaemia. A prospective randomised controlled study comparing the 1-year results of vascular surgery and percutaneous transluminal angioplasty (PTA). Eur J Vasc Surg, 1991. 5(5): p. 517-22.

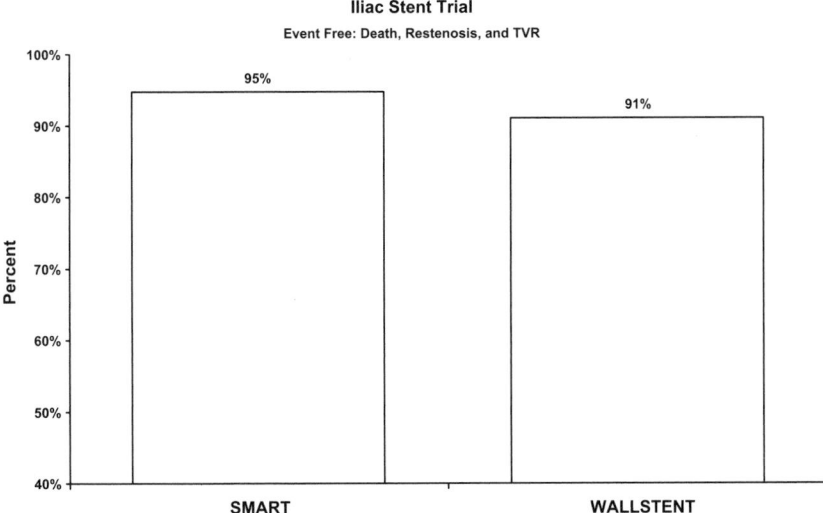

Figure 6-4. CRISP trial: One year outcome comparing nitinol (SMART) and stainless steel (Wallstent) iliac stents. Ponec, D., et al., The Nitinol SMART stent vs Wallstent for suboptimal iliac artery angioplasty: CRISP-US trial results. J Vasc Interv Radiol, 2004. 15(9): p. 911-8.

stent placement with self-expanding stents have been reported in patients following failed or suboptimal angioplasty in iliac lesions (21). Vorwerk and colleagues demonstrated excellent outcomes for provisional iliac stent placement in aorto-iliac lesions. They reported primary patency at 1 year of 95%, 2 years of 88%, and 4 years of 82% in 118 treated lesions (22).

Primary versus provisional iliac stent placement was compared in a randomized trial. Pressure gradients across the lesions after primary stent placement (5.8 ± 4.7 mmHg) were significantly lower than after balloon angioplasty alone (8.9 ± 6.8 mmHg), but not after provisional stenting (5.9 ± 3.6 mmHg) in the PTA group (23). The procedural success rate, defined as a post-procedural gradient less than 10 mmHg, revealed no difference between the two treatment strategies, (primary stenting = 81% versus PTA plus provisional stenting = 89%). By employing a provisional stenting strategy, stent placement was avoided in 63% of the lesions, and still achieved an equivalent hemodynamic result compared to primary stenting.

Endovascular Therapy for Femoral-Popliteal Disease

Claudication

Patients selected for PTA should have a significant limitation of their lifestyle or be limited at work and/or have failed to respond to conservative therapy (medication and supervised exercise) with a favorable risk-to-benefit ratio for intervention (1). There have been only a small number of trials comparing outcomes of medical therapy, PTA, or surgery for claudicants with femoral-popliteal arterial disease. Using a decision-analysis model to determine the cost-effectiveness and quality-of-life outcomes in patients treated for claudication demonstrates that PTA, performed whenever feasible, is more effective than exercise alone, with a cost-effectiveness ratio within the generally accepted range (Figure 6-5) (24). For claudicants, where durability of the procedure is the key to success, if the 5-year vessel patency is = 30%, then PTA will be superior to surgery (25).

Consistent with this strategy, a large prospective, matched cohort study of 526 patients with intermittent claudication found significant advantages for a revascularization strategy (surgery or PTA) compared to medical therapy (26). Revascularization patients had functional improvement superior to medically managed patients, including measurements of physical function, bodily pain, and walking distance. The highest ABI measurements correlated with the best clinical improvement, suggesting that the degree of revascularization was related to a successful outcome. Exercise therapy compared to PTA in claudicants using a meta-analysis found no difference for quality-of-life measures at 3 and 6 months but did show that functional capacity (ABI improvement) improved more with PTA than with exercise therapy (27).

There are two randomized trials showing equivalent hemodynamic improvement and patency for PTA compared to surgical bypass in patients with femoral-popliteal lesions (Figures 6-2 and 6-3) (13,14). There was no significant difference between the two groups at follow-up for study-related deaths, amputations, and late interventions. The authors concluded that in

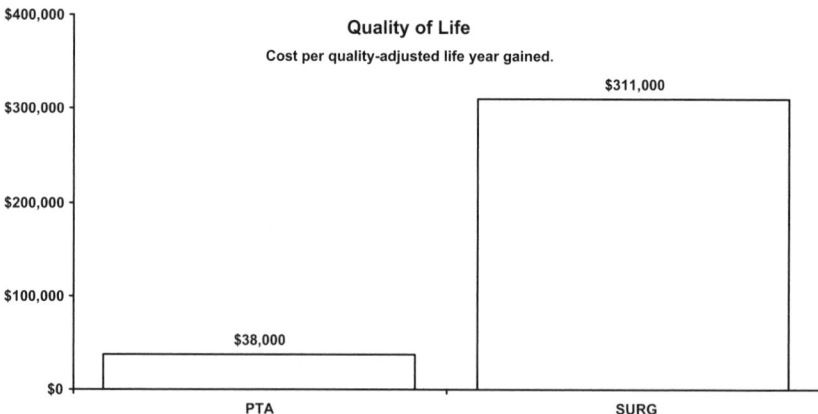

Figure 6-5. Cost effectiveness of PTA vs Surgery for claudication. de Vries, S.O., et al., *Intermittent claudication: cost-effectiveness of revascularization versus exercise therapy.* Radiology, 2002. 222(1): p. 25-36.

lesions that are amenable to either angioplasty or surgery, angioplasty should be chosen first for its lower morbidity and cost and equivalent long-term results (13,14).

A European study reported the results of a randomized trial of PTA or medical therapy for patients with single-leg claudication (28). At the 6-month follow-up assessment, the balloon angioplasty group could walk farther before the onset of symptoms, and had a significantly higher ankle-brachial index (ABI). The most important benefit for the PTA group was improved vessel patency, as only 3.6% of patients in the PTA group had developed an occlusion compared to 41.2% in the medically treated group (P <0.001).

The status of the distal run-off bed affects the long-term success of PTA in the femoral-popliteal vessels. In one study of 370 patients undergoing angioplasty for lower limb ischemia, patients with <1 vessel run-off had a 3-year patency of only 25%, compared with 78% in patients with 2- or 3-vessel runoff (29). Minar and colleagues analyzed restenosis at 2 years in 207 patients following successful femoropopliteal angioplasty and used a multivariate analysis to assess variables affecting restenosis (Table 6-4) (30). Femoral-popliteal PTA results have improved over time with reported patency rates of 87% at 1 year, 69% at 3 years, and 55% at 5 years in contemporary series (31). The long-term patency of femoral-popliteal angioplasty depends on clinical as well as anatomic variables (29,32,33). Clinical factors that negatively affect the long-term patency of PTA include female sex, diabetes, and the presence of rest pain or threatened limb loss. Technical factors that correlate with long-term failure of angioplasty include longer lesion length, multiple versus single lesions, lesion eccentricity, and a poor angiographic appearance post-angioplasty.

PTA has a procedural success rate between 70% and 97% for femoral-popliteal atherosclerotic lesions, being higher for stenoses than for total occlusions (34,35). The current evidence-based recommendation regarding femoral-popliteal artery stents is to use them in a "provisional" strategy. Stents should be reserved for salvage of a failed balloon angioplasty result in femoral-popliteal arteries. An exception to this may favor stent placement in patients with longer lesions, occlusions, and those with limb-threatening ischemia where there is evidence of superior stent performance compared to balloon angioplasty (36).

Self-expanding stents are preferred in femoral and popliteal arteries because of the risk of stent compression from external trauma. Early non-randomized clinical series suggested that superficial femoral artery (SFA) stent placement could be accomplished with a very high primary success rate, and that the restenosis rates were the lowest in the larger diameter arteries, shorter lesions, and with fewer stents placed (20,21). The US Food and Drug Administration approved the IntraCoil stent (Sulzer, Minneapolis, MN) in 2001 for the primary treatment of symptomatic atherosclerotic disease in the femoral-popliteal arteries. This was based on data from 266 patients entered into a pivotal US randomized trial. Patients were included in the trial if they had 1) symptomatic leg ischemia and they were candidates for balloon angioplasty, 2) stenoses = 15 cm long or occlusions = 12 cm long, and 3) the target lesion was proximal to the tibial artery bifurcation. At 9 months there was no difference in target-lesion revascularization (TLR) between the stent group (14.3%) and the balloon group (16.1%, p = NS); however, there was an advantage for the stent in the longer lesion lengths (Figures 6-6 and 6-7) (37).

A meta-analysis compared SFA stent placement to balloon angioplasty between 1993 and 2000 (36). A total of 923 balloon dilations and 473 stent placements were compared. In contrast to results of SFA balloon angioplasty, long-term vessel patency after stent placement was minimally affected by the clinical indication or the lesion morphology. However, compared to SFA balloon angioplasty, stent placement did yield better results in patients with occlusions and critical limb ischemia (36).

The role of primary stent placement in SFA revascularization remains controversial. The SFA is subject to repeated longitudinal stretching, external compression, torsion, and flexion; these stresses may predispose to stent fractures, which have been linked to restenosis (38). Early randomized trials comparing PTA with stent placement for SFA lesions failed to demonstrate an advantage for stent placement compared to PTA with bail-out stent placement (36,39).

The most recent randomized controlled trial of primary verus provisional stenting demonstrated significantly higher patency rates at 1 year for SFA stent placement compared to PTA with bail-out stent placement (Figure 6-8); the stent group also had significantly better walking distance and ABI measurements at 1 year. The low-risk nature of SFA intervention was

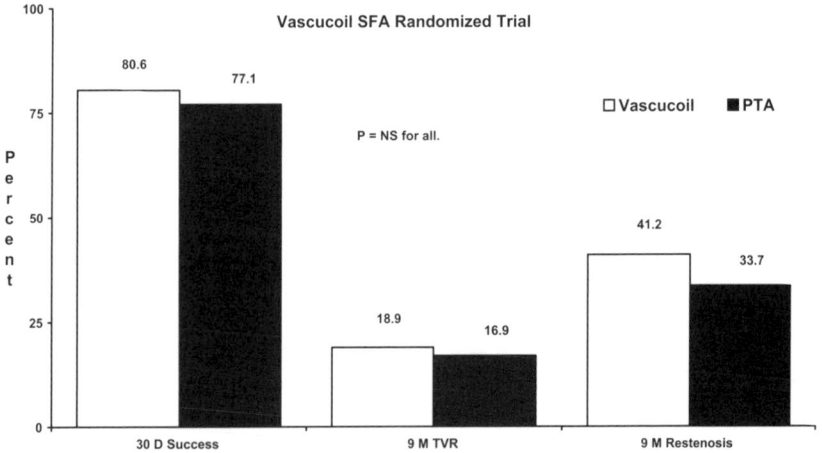

Figure 6-6. Vascucoil SFA Randomized Trial (N = 266).

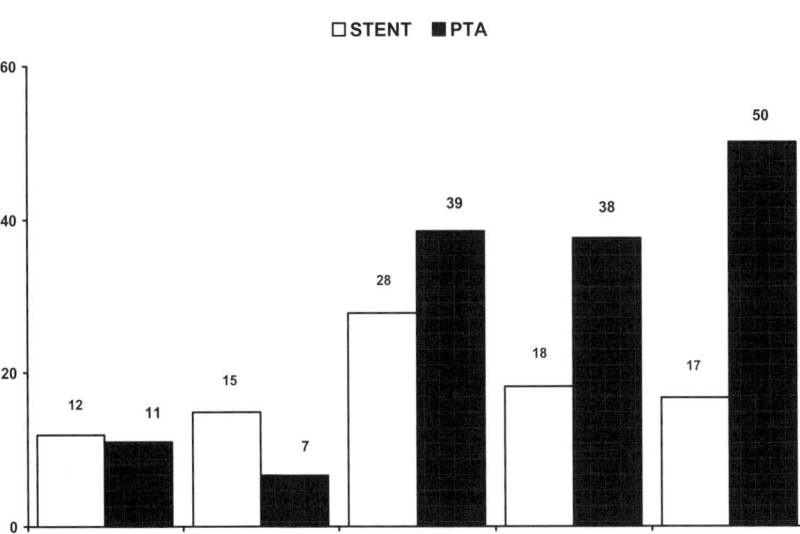

Figure 6-7. SFA Restenosis by lesion length for the Vascucoil randomized trial. United States Food and Drug Adminstration, Center for Devices and Radiological Health, Intracoil® Self-Expanding Peripheral Stent P000033: Summary of Safety and Effectiveness. 2002.

demonstrated in this trial, as there were no major complications in either group (40).

Critical Limb Ischemia

The Bypass versus Angioplasty in Severe Ischemia of the Leg (BASIL) trial compared percutaneous transluminal angioplasty (PTA) to surgery in 452 patients with rest pain, ulceration, or gangrene of the leg secondary to infra-inguinal disease (41). The primary end-point, amputation-free survival, was similar for PTA and surgery at 1 year (71% vs. 68%, p = NS) and 3 years (52% vs. 57%, P = NS). Although there was no significant difference in mortality between the groups at 30 days, surgery was associated with a higher post-procedure morbidity. The mortality within the entire cohort over the course of the study (5.5 years) was 37%, which underscores the poor prognosis due to cardiovascular diseases of patients who present with CLI. During the initial hospitalization, almost three times as many patients treated with surgery required admission to the intensive care or high-dependency unit compared to those treated with angioplasty (27% vs. 7.5%), which resulted in the cost of hospitalization being higher in the surgical group (Table 6-5).

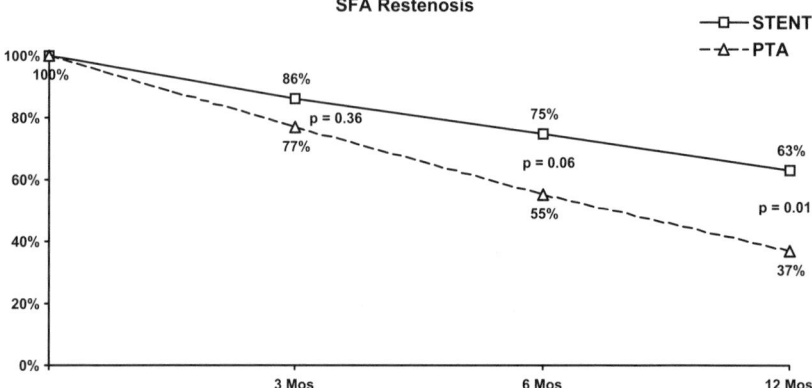

Figure 6-8. SFA restenosis for drug-eluting stents vs bare metal stents. Schillinger, M., et al., *Balloon angioplasty versus implantation of nitinol stents in the superficial femoral artery.* N Engl J Med, 2006. 354(18): p. 1879-88.

Table 6-5.   Overview of Therapies Used for the Treatment of Critical Limb Ischemia: Cost of Devices and Reported Outcomes*

Device/Technique	Cost per Device	Technical Success Rate (%)	One-Year Primary Patency Rate (%)	One-Year Limb Salvage Rate (%)
PTA	$260	89-93	59-79	81-92
Bare metal stent	$1100	96-100	62-86	89-97
Drug-eluting stent (below-knee only)	$3200	100	92 (6-month)	100 (6-month)
Cutting balloon	$1000	100 (20% stent usage)	NA	89.5
Cryoplasty catheter (PolarCath)	$2200	NA	NA	NA
Excimer laser catheter (CLiRPath)	$1600	86 (45% stent usage)	NA	93 (6-month)
		84 (80% stent usage)	NA	72 (1-year)
Atherectomy catheter (SilverHawk)	$4200	99 (17% stent usage)	NA	80 (6-month)
		87 (5% stent usage)	62	86 (1-year)

*Cost is average per single device or catheter and does not include price of additional devices or equipment, e.g., stents. Reported success rates vary by disease location; range includes success rates for the entire limb. Only studies with 20 or more patients are included. Unpublished data (including presentations and manufacturer-supplied data) have been excluded. Data combines results from studies of nitinol and stainless steel stents in lower-extremity interventions, as well as coronary stent implantation in infra-popliteal locations. DES data only includes 6-month outcomes following sirolimus eluting stents implantation in infra-popliteal locations. Different values are listed because of significant differences in % stent usage and duration of follow-up.

PTA was associated with higher immediate failure rate and 12-month re-intervention rates in the BASIL study. This did not affect the patients' candidacy for a second percutaneous procedure or subsequent surgery. Post hoc analysis demonstrated that surgery was associated with a lower rate of amputation and death (hazard ratio 0.34, CI 0.17-0.71) in patients alive at 2 years with the treated limb intact. The authors suggested that the healthier patients, i.e. those with a life expectancy exceeding 2 years, may benefit from surgical intervention as initial therapy for limb-threatening ischemia. BASIL demonstrated that endovascular therapy and surgery were comparable as first-line therapy for CLI, but that PTA was less expensive and did not preclude subsequent treatment with surgery. PTA should be chosen first if a patient is a candidate for either procedure, particularly if the patient's life expectancy is less than 2 years (41,42).

Clinical risk factors associated with poor outcomes following iliac interventions in CLI patients include female gender and chronic renal insufficiency (43). In this non-randomized series, 42% of patients were treated with primary stent placement (at the operators discretion), while the remainder were treated with PTA followed by provisional (bail-out) stent placement. The technical success rate for all procedures was 96%, and primary stent patency rates were 90% at 1 year, 74% at 3 years, and 69% at 5 years. Patency rates were lower in women (RR 5.1, P = 0.002) and those with renal insufficiency (Cr >1.6) (RR 6.6, P = 0.01).

Therapy for Tibial-Peroneal (Below-Knee) Disease

Below-knee angioplasty has been generally reserved for cases of threatened limb loss critical limb ischemia because of the technical difficulty using conventional peripheral angioplasty equipment in these vessels, and the fear of potential limb loss should a complication occur. Early published experience with PTA demonstrated the feasibility of a percutaneous approach, documenting procedural success rates >80% for tibioperoneal angioplasty (44,45). The adoption and use of coronary angioplasty equipment improved the results of below-knee intervention. In 111 patients with tibioperoneal angioplasty for claudication (47%), tissue loss (27%), or rest pain (26%), Dorros and co-workers (46) reported a primary success rate of 90% for all lesions, including a 99% success rate for stenoses and a 65% success rate for occlusions. At the time of hospital discharge, 95% of the patients were symptomatically improved.

Two more recent trials have demonstrated the efficacy and attractiveness of an initial percutaneous approach to selected patients with critical limb ischemia and infrapopliteal vascular disease (47,48). The limb-salvage rate in these patients treated with PTA after 2 to 5 years range from 85% to 91%. This evidence supports the contention that angioplasty of the tibioperoneal vessels should not necessarily be reserved for limb-salvage situations;

however, caution is still advised in patient selection because the surgical options are limited if angioplasty fails.

Optimal treatment of infra-popliteal disease requires appropriate patient and lesion selection for treatment. Focal stenoses have the best outcomes, with fewer than five separate lesions associated with a higher success rate. The goal of therapy is relief of rest pain, healing of ulcers, and avoiding amputation, and not necessarily long-term vessel patency. When trying to heal ischemic ulcers, the basic principle is that it takes more oxygenated blood flow to heal a wound than to maintain tissue integrity (47). Recent clinical trials suggest that percutaneous therapy can result in long-term limb salvage in more than 80% of patients and should be considered the current standard of treatment in patients with limb-threatening ischemia who are candidates for endovascular intervention (47,48).

Urgent Endovascular Therapy for Patients with Peripheral Arterial Disease

Critical limb ischemia (CLI) occurs when reduced arterial perfusion results in rest pain and/or tissue breakdown in the lower extremities. It is associated with a high cardiovascular morbidity and mortality: as many as 24% of patients with CLI will die within the first year after presentation (3,4). The optimal treatment for CLI is prompt revascularization utilizing endovascular intervention or vascular bypass surgery. Percutaneous transluminal angioplasty (PTA) is the initial therapy of choice for CLI in patients who are candidates for either surgery or endovascular therapy to avoid the additional morbidity associated with vascular surgery (1,2). Endovascular intervention does not preclude the possibility of subsequent surgery, and in fact there is often a role for both modalities. In patients who are poor candidates for surgery, such as those with poor distal targets, those who lack adequate saphenous vein for bypass grafting, and those with severe comorbidities, endovascular therapy may offer the only opportunity for limb salvage.

The therapeutic goal in patients presenting with CLI is to re-establish pulsatile, straight-line flow to the distal extremity. This usually involves treatment of multiple arterial segments at the same setting. Establishment of uninterrupted flow to at least one infrapopliteal vessel, i.e. the anterior/posterior tibial or peroneal arteries, is a prerequisite for wound healing.

Adjuvant Device Therapies Used for Endovascular Therapy

The endovascular treatment of lower-extremity lesions with angioplasty and stents is associated with technical success rates that vary from 86% to 100% (36). The most common reason for immediate failure is inability to cross the lesion or to gain re-entry into the distal lumen. Late failure most often occurs due to in-stent restenosis as a result of intimal hyperplasia. Stent fracture accelerates restenosis by promoting intimal hyperplasia, and some degree of stent disruption may be detected in as many as 24% cases following femoral artery stent placement (38). The risk of stent fracture, and risk of restenosis, is directly related to length of the stented segment. Several adjunctive therapies and devices have been introduced to improve procedure success and late patency. As previously noted, there is no Level I comparative data to support routine use of these devices during endovascular revascularization (Figure 6-9).

Cutting Balloon Angioplasty

The cutting balloon catheter (Boston Scientific Corporation, Natick, MA) is a device in which razor blades are embedded on the exterior of the balloon. These atherotomes, which are arranged longitudinally, are intended to score the plaque surface during balloon expansion. Proponents of the device claim that cutting balloons are less traumatic to the vessel wall and

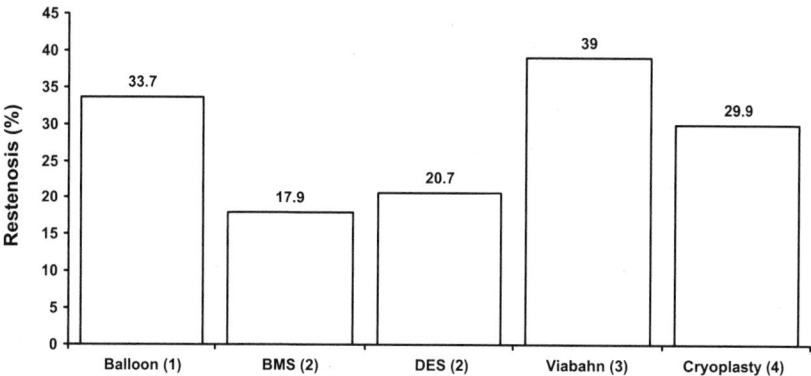

Figure 6-9. SFA restenosis for multiple devices ranging from 9 to 18 months of follow-up. BMS = bare metal stent, DES = drug eluting stent, Cryo = cryoplasty 1) Vascucoil Stent vs PTA; randomized trial, from the FDA submission (United States Food and Drug Administration, Center for Devices and Radiological Health, Intracoil® Self-Expanding Peripheral Stent P000033: Summary of Safety and Effectiveness. 2002). 2) SIROCCO II randomized trial,18 month ultrasound restenosis data. (Duda, S.H., et al., *Sirolimus-eluting versus bare nitinol stent for obstructive superficial femoral artery disease: the SIROCCO II trial.* J Vasc Interv Radiol, 2005. 16(3): p. 331-8.) 3) Gore VIABAHN vs PTA, randomized trial, from the FDA submission. (*United States Food and Drug Administration, Center for Devices and Radiological Health: GORE VIABAHN™ Endoprosthesis - P040037.* 2005 (cited; Available from: http://www.fda.gov/cdrh/mda/docs/p040037.html) 4) Cryoplasty registry (Laird, J., et al., *Cryoplasty for the treatment of femoropopliteal arterial disease: results of a prospective, multicenter registry.* J Vasc Interv Radiol, 2005. 16(8): p. 1067-73.)

limit the extent of dissection following angioplasty, but this has yet to be demonstrated in a convincing manner (Figure 6-10) (49,50). The atherotomes make the device bulky compared to standard angioplasty balloons, and data from cutting balloon angioplasty (CBA) in the coronaries suggests that cutting balloons may actually predispose to vessel perforations (51).

In one study, infrainguinal CBA was performed in 73 patients with limb ischemia, the vast majority of whom (71%) presented with rest pain or threatened limbs. The authors reported a technical success rate of 100% and a limb-salvage rate of 89.5% at 1 year (49). The results of CBA were suboptimal in 20% of subjects, and bail-out stents were required to treat severe intimal dissection or a residual stenosis in these patients. These outcomes were similar to those of PTA with provisional stent placement in the current literature but at a much higher cost (52).

Cryoplasty

The PolarCath (Boston Scientific Corporation, Natick, MA), is a device that combines balloon angioplasty with the delivery of cold thermal energy to the vessel wall. It consists of a specialized balloon catheter attached to a source of pressurized nitrous oxide (NO) that is used to simultaneously inflate and cool the balloon to sub-zero temperatures. Proponents of the technique have suggested that application of cryoplasty leads to apoptosis and reduced restenosis, but a recent study in humans showed no difference for cryoplasty compared to PTA for release of the growth factors and cytokines that initiate neo-intimal hyperplasia (53). Clinical data show that outcomes

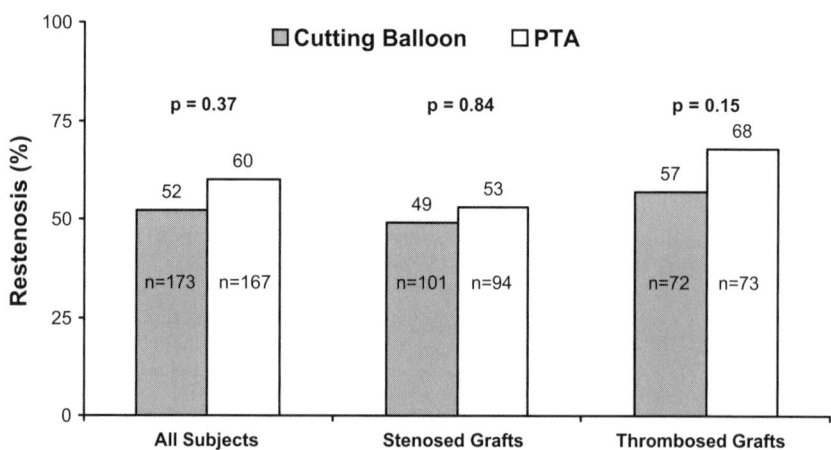

Figure 6-10. Cutting balloon vs PTA for SFA lesions.

following cryoplasty in claudicants are no better than the results that may be expected with conventional balloon angioplasty (Figure 6-11) (54,55).

Excimer Laser Assisted Angioplasty

Excimer laser-assisted (ELA) angioplasty was introduced as an adjunct to endovascular interventions over two decades ago. The CLiRPath catheter (Spectranetics, Inc., Colorado Springs, CO) is the only unit to be approved by the FDA for use in the peripheral vasculature. This device uses excited dimers, hence the term "excimer," to generate short, intense pulses of ultraviolet (UV) light (56,57). The proposed mechanism by which the laser debulks atheromatous plaque is "photoablation," i.e. destruction of plaque material by photochemical energy contained within the UV pulses (58). Successful recanalization using excimer laser does not eliminate the need for subsequent balloon angioplasty because the diameter of even the largest catheter (2.5 mm) is smaller than the typical diameter of the femoral arteries where it is commonly used (Figure 6-12).

To date there have been no randomized trials comparing ELA to conventional angioplasty for CLI. The Laser Angioplasty for Critical Limb Ischemia (LACI) study was a non-randomized, multicenter registry in which 145 patients were treated using ELA (59). Procedural success, defined as a residual stenosis of <50%, was achieved in 86% of cases; angioplasty was needed in 96% and stents were used in 45% of limbs. These results showed that ELA, in conjunction with PTA and provisional stent placement, could be used successfully to treat patients with CLI. However, the trial failed to

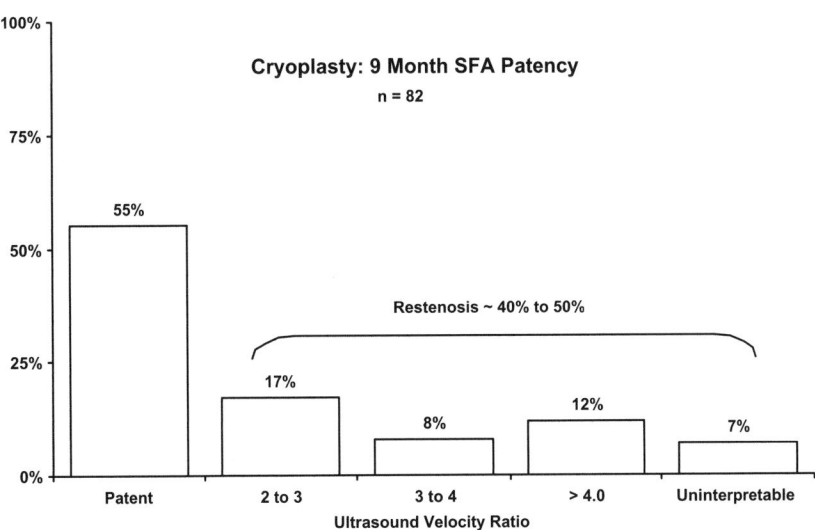

Figure 6-11. Cryocath and 9 month duplex ultrasound velocity ratio results.

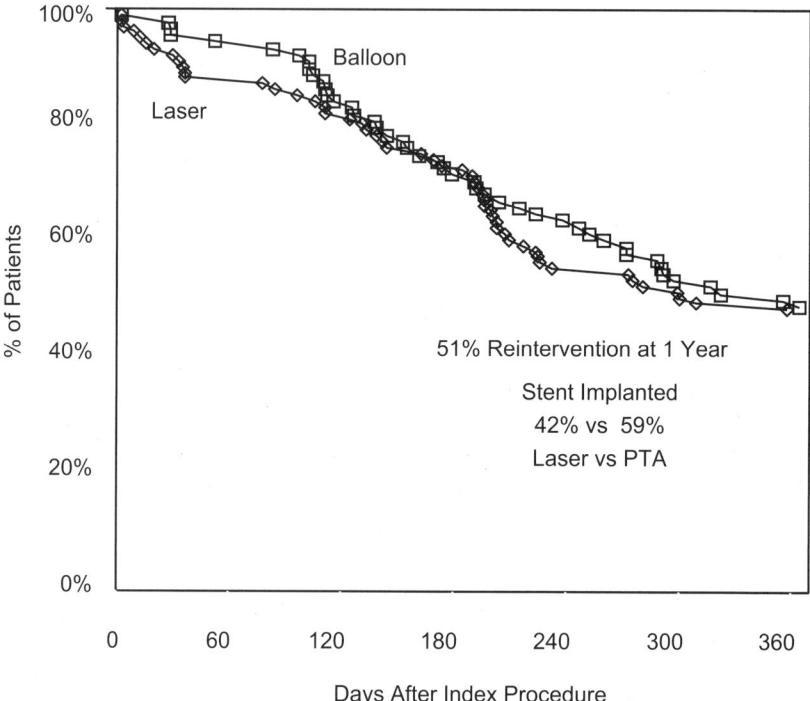

Figure 6-12.   Freedom from reintervention is not different for LASER or PTA.

demonstrate that use of ELA improved clinical outcomes when compared to PTA and provisional stent placement, or that it was more cost-effective.

Atherectomy

The concept of plaque excision as an adjunct, or alternative, to angioplasty has been around for over a decade, and recent years have seen a renewed interest in atherectomy for the treatment of peripheral arteries. The most commonly used device is the SilverHawk Excision System (Fox Hollow Technologies, Redwood City, CA), which is a directional atherectomy catheter. Plaque is shaved off as the atherectomy blade at the tip of the device rotates. At present there is no randomized data to show that this device is actually associated with lower rates of restenosis or of distal embolization.

Excisional atherectomy as an alternative to surgery or angioplasty with stent placement was reported in 69 patients (160 lesions) with CLI, i.e. rest pain or threatened limb loss (60). All patients were treated with the SilverHawk atherectomy catheter, and adjunctive therapy with PTA or stents was required in 17% of cases. After 6 months, 66% of patients had improved clinically, whereas 13% required an amputation, 14% had died, and 7% underwent target vessel revascularization. The patency rates and limb-salvage rates with excisional atherectomy reported in this study were similar, but not superior, to results of other endovascular therapies that have been reported elsewhere.

Bare Metal Stents

Self-expanding stents have the ability to regain their original configuration after compression. This property, called "shape memory," has made these stents a popular choice for implantation in arteries that are tortuous and/or are repeatedly subject to external forces, particularly the lower-extremity arteries outside the protective barrier of the axial skeleton. Self-expanding stents also lend themselves to tapering and tortuous vessels such as are found in the iliac arteries. They are made of nitinol or stainless steel, and there are comparative studies in the iliac arteries to show that they are equal in performance. The major disadvantage of self-expanding stents is the operator is never absolutely sure how long the stent will be once it is expanded. For this reason, when precision is necessary, we use balloon expandable stents, which are more predictable. Balloon-expandable stents also have more radial strength to resist compressive forces from heavily calcified arteries.

Drug-Eluting Stents

Drug-coated stents (DES) have revolutionized coronary intervention by markedly reducing the restenosis rate by suppressing intimal hyperplasia. However, the results for peripheral drug-coated stents have not been encouraging (Figure 6-9). Peripheral drug-coated stents (sirolimus) were compared to bare metal (nitinol) self-expanding stents in a randomized trial that included 93 patients with claudication. All stents were implanted within the superficial femoral artery, and patients followed clinically and with ultrasound. After 2 years, the duplex-derived patency rates for DES and BMS were almost identical: 22.9% in the sirolimus versus 21.1% in the bare stent group (61). The fact that sirolimus-coated stents failed to show superiority over bare metal stents in this study can be attributed to very low restenosis rates seen with BMS. Although DES are not used for femoro-popliteal lesions, their role in infra-inguinal interventions is still being investigated. As noted above, coronary DES have been successfully implanted in tibial and peroneal arteries to treat critical limb ischemia (62,63).

Stent Grafts

A stent-graft consists of a self-expanding stent covered by a porous tube of polytetrafluoroethylene (PTFE). Though PTFE-covered stents were originally designed to exclude arterial aneurysms and perforations, they are increasingly being used to treat atherosclerotic disease within the femoral arteries. One such device is the Gore Viabahn Endoprosthesis (W.L. Gore and Associates Inc., Flagstaff, AZ), which was approved for femoral artery implantation by the FDA in 2005 (Figures 6-13 and 6-14) (64). No large randomized trials evaluating the Viabahn stent-graft have been published to date. In data submitted to the FDA, which included 241 claudicants, the reported 1-year primary patency rates were 51% vs. 45% in patients randomized to stent-grafts or PTA, respectively. Thrombosis and distal embolization were major complications of the device and were almost twice as prevalent when compared to conventional PTA (65). Though a few small, nonrandomized studies have shown that stent-grafts can be used successfully, larger comparative trials are needed to establish the clinical efficacy and safety of stent-grafts in this population.

Bioabsorbable Stents

Metal stents made from stainless steel and nitinol become permanently implanted in the arterial wall following deployment, which is the mechanism by which they provide mechanical support to the vessel wall. However, this permanently alters the compliance of the blood vessel. In addition there has been concern that the continued presence of stents causes a prolonged inflammatory response at the site of implantation, predisposing to late problems such as delayed restenosis and thrombosis (66). Bioabsorbable stents, which are stents that dissolve following implantation, were developed to ad-

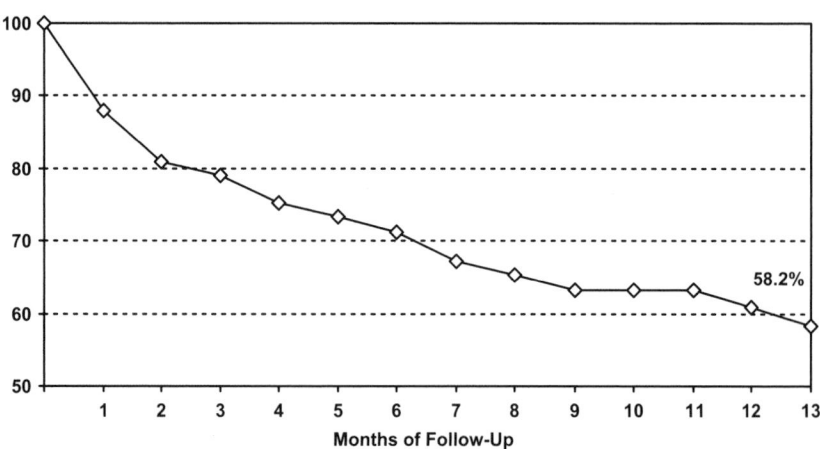

Figure 6-13. Covered Stent-Graft SFA (Hemobahn) Primary Patency. Acute thrombosis = 24 hrs in 6.8% (n = 4). Acute thrombosis = 24 hrs in 6.8% (n = 4). Bray PJ, et al. J Endovasc Ther 2003;10:619-28.

SFA 12 Month Primary Patency

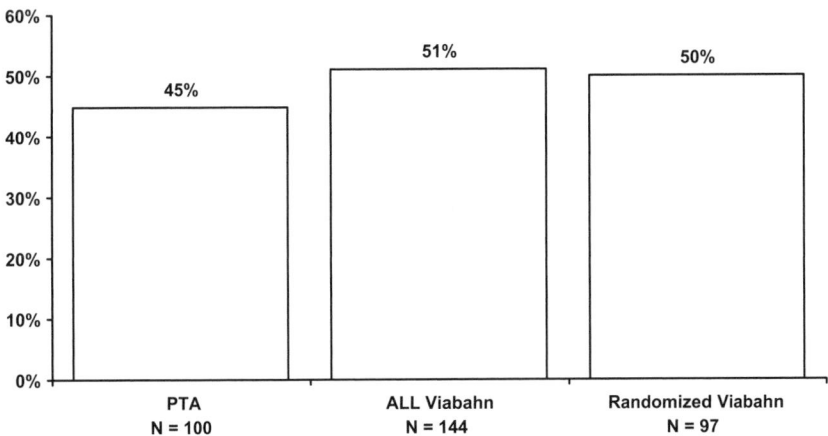

Figure 6-14. SFA 12 month primary patency rate for Gore Viabahn® vs PTA. United States Food and Drug Adminstration, Center for Devices and Radiological Health: GORE VIABAHN™ Endoprosthesis - P040037. 2005 (cited; Available from: http://www.fda.gov/cdrh/mda/docs/p040037.html

dress these issues (67). Bioabsorbable stents made from magnesium have been successfully implanted in humans, and were used to treat 20 patients with critical limb ischemia in one small study (68). All stents were placed in either the tibial or peroneal arteries, and stent absorption was confirmed by ultrasonography during follow-up. At 6 months, the limb salvage and duplex-derived primary patency rates were 94% and 79%, respectively. Though these results are interesting, larger studies are needed to better define the role of bioabsorbable stents in lower-extremity interventions.

Brachytherapy with Gamma Irradiation (^{192}Ir)

Local delivery of radiation therapy has demonstrated mixed results for reducing restenosis after PTA in de novo SFA lesions (69,70). There is evidence that it is effective in reducing recurrence when used in conjunction with PTA for restenosis lesions (71). In de novo SFA lesions, an increased rate of early thrombosis (17%) without improvement in restenosis was observed in the brachytherapy with stent arm (72). Endovascular brachytherapy has suffered from limited availability largely as a result of coronary DES completely displacing coronary brachytherapy. Endovascular brachytherapy with gamma sources requires extensive shielding and transportation of the patient from the cath lab to a radiation therapy suite, which is cumbersome. A novel solution, which deserves further study, has been external beam radiation. In a dose-response trial, positive results were seen with a single treatment session delivering 14 Gy to SFA lesions after PTA only (73).

Gene Therapy

The use of gene or cellular therapies for lower-extremity ischemia has demonstrated mixed results between the basic science laboratory and clinical medicine. At this time, larger controlled clinical trials are needed to establish a role for these therapies (74-77) (See chapter 8).

Adjuvant Medical Therapies Used for Endovascular Therapy

All patients with established peripheral vascular disease should be treated with aspirin (81 mg daily). Aspirin therapy should be initiated at the time of the pre-procedure evaluation if not already established. At present there is no evidence to suggest that the additional use of other antiplatelet agents, such as clopidogrel or ticlopidine, improves procedural success rates or decreases complications. Dual anti-platelet therapy is therefore optional in patients undergoing endovascular revascularization, though further investigation may be warranted in this population, which is characterized by a high incidence of adverse cardiovascular events as noted previously. Clopidogrel is the drug of choice in patients who are intolerant of or resistant to aspirin.

Patients undergoing percutaneous revascularization must be anticoagulated for the duration of the procedure. Heparin is the most commonly used anti-coagulant in the catheterization laboratory. There is no evidence to support the routine use of other anticoagulants, such as bivalirudin, for lower-extremity interventions. Bivalirudin, which is considerably more expensive than heparin, should only be used for patients who cannot be treated with heparin, e.g. those with heparin-induced thrombocytopenia. Chronic anti-coagulation with warfarin is not indicated because of the increased risk of bleeding and lack of evidence demonstrating efficacy in these patients.

Follow-Up in Patients Treated with Endovascular Therapy

Patients with critical limb ischemia need to be followed closely after percutaneous therapy. Not only does this give the interventionalist or surgeon an opportunity to monitor the patient's response to the revascularization, it also allows early identification of recurrent problems and of treatment failure (78). This is particularly important in patients likely to require multiple procedures for sustained benefit: diabetics, patients with multivessel disease, and those with prior procedures (79). The importance of a multidisciplinary team approach cannot be over-stressed in this regard. The interventionalist performing the procedure should work closely with a vascular medicine specialist and the patient's primary care physician.

During the initial period of healing, the patient should be seen every 3 to 4 weeks, typically until the foot lesions have completely healed. Each visit should include a thorough cardiovascular evaluation, including blood pressure and heart rate measurement, as well as visual examination of the extremities. Proximal and distal pulses should be palpated and diligently documented. Ankle-brachial indices should be recorded prior to hospital discharge, and then in the office once every 6 to 12 months. The office visit should be used as an opportunity to address risk factors for development of other types of cardiovascular diseases. Hypertension, hyperlipidemia, and diabetes mellitus, if present, should be treated aggressively. Smoking cessation should be emphasized and referral to a smoking cessation program should be offered. Once healing is complete, the frequency of visits may be decreased.

Exercise ABI testing should be performed once yearly, or sooner if the patient develops worsening or recurrent symptoms. Lower-extremity ultrasonography should be performed at 3 months after the procedure, and then every 6 to 12 months thereafter. Ultrasonography should be repeated sooner if the patient develops symptoms. Computed tomography and magnetic resonance imaging are not routinely indicated, and should be reserved for symptomatic patients, those with an abnormal or non-diagnostic ultrasound, or those in whom a repeat procedure is being contemplated.

Summary

Endovascular revascularization is indicated for symptomatic patients who do not respond adequately to pharmacotherapy and supervised exercise therapy, and for those who present critical limb ischemia (i.e., rest pain, non-healing ulcers, or gangrene). There are no absolute contraindications to endovascular intervention, and percutaneous transluminal angioplasty (PTA) is the initial therapy of choice in symptomatic patients with PAD because it avoids the morbidity associated with vascular surgery. Treatment of claudication is directed towards symptom relief and restoration of limb function, whereas treatment of critical limb ischemia is directed towards limb salvage, i.e. avoiding amputation. Endovascular therapy may offer the only opportunity for symptom-relief and limb salvage in patients who are poor candidates for surgery.

Optimal treatment of infra-popliteal disease requires appropriate patient and lesion selection for treatment. Patency rates following angioplasty are highest for the iliac arteries, and decrease with distal disease sites. Other anatomic criteria that affect outcomes following revascularization include increasing lesion length, the presence of multiple lesions, chronic total occlusions, and the coexistence of "inflow" and "outflow" disease. Clinical features that affect outcomes include functional status, the presence of diabetes, renal insufficiency, and smoking.

The availability of endovascular stents has significantly extended the anatomic subset of patients that may be considered candidates for percutaneous revascularization, particularly for longer lesions and occlusions. Several stent technologies have been introduced in an effort to prolong the durability of percutaneous interventions by minimizing late stent failure from restenosis.

The current evidence-based guidelines recommend primary stent placement within the iliac arteries. Angioplasty with provisional stent placement is the treatment of choice in femoral-popliteal arteries. Self-expanding stents are preferred in femoral and popliteal arteries because of the risk of stent compression and fracture from external trauma. Brachytherapy with gamma irradiation has demonstrated mixed results for reducing restenosis after PTA in SFA lesions. Below-knee angioplasty has been generally reserved for cases of threatened limb loss critical limb ischemia. These vessels have been safely treated with both bare-metal and drug-eluting stents, though there is no data to support routine stent placement at these sites.

Several adjunctive therapies and devices have been introduced to improve procedure success and late patency following endovascular revascularization in the lower extremities. Given the high cost of many of the devices, and lack of randomized data showing superior outcomes with adjunctive therapies compared to conventional angioplasty, the use of these technologies should be limited to patients who fail conventional endovascular techniques and are facing the prospect of imminent limb loss.

All patients with established peripheral vascular disease should be treated with aspirin, or clopidogrel if they cannot take aspirin. Patients with severe PAD need to be followed closely after endovascular therapy, and periodic surveillance is essential to identify restenosis as early as possible. A multi-disciplinary team approach is essential in this regard.

REFERENCES

1. Hirsch AT, et al. ACC/AHA 2005 guidelines for the management of patients with peripheral arterial disease (lower extremity, renal, mesenteric, and abdominal aortic): executive summary a collaborative report from the American Association for Vascular Surgery/Society for Vascular Surgery, Society for Cardiovascular Angiography and Interventions, Society for Vascular Medicine and Biology, Society of Interventional Radiology, and the ACC/AHA Task Force on Practice Guidelines (Writing Committee to Develop Guidelines for the Management of Patients With Peripheral Arterial Disease) endorsed by the American Association of Cardiovascular and Pulmonary Rehabilitation; National Heart, Lung, and Blood Institute; Society for Vascular Nursing; TransAtlantic Inter-Society Consensus; and Vascular Disease Foundation. J Am Coll Cardiol. 2006; 47:1239-312.

2. Norgren L, et al. Inter-Society Consensus for the Management of Peripheral Arterial Disease (TASC II). Eur J Vasc Endovasc Surg. 2007;33(Suppl 1):S1-75.

3. Barani J, et al. Cardiac function, inflammatory mediators and mortality in critical limb ischemia. Angiology. 2006;57:437-44.

4. **Barani J, et al**. Suboptimal treatment of risk factor for atherosclerosis in critical limb ischemia. Int Angiol. 2005;24:59-63.
5. **Dormandy JA, Rutherford RB**. Management of peripheral arterial disease (PAD). TASC Working Group. TransAtlantic Inter-Society Concensus (TASC). J Vasc Surg. 2000;31(1 Pt 2):S1-S296.
6. **Johnston KW**. Iliac arteries: reanalysis of results of balloon angioplasty. Radiology. 1993; 186:207-12.
7. **Jeans WD, et al**. Randomized trial of laser-assisted passage through occluded femoropopliteal arteries. Br J Radiol. 1990;63:19-21.
8. **Tegtmeyer CJ, et al**. Results and complications of angioplasty in aortoiliac disease. Circulation. 1991;83(2 Suppl):I53-60.
9. **Casarella WJ**. Noncoronary angioplasty. Curr Probl Cardiol. 1986;11:141-74.
10. **Gallino A, et al**. Percutaneous transluminal angioplasty of the arteries of the lower limbs: a 5 year follow-up. Circulation. 1984;70:619-23.
11. **Johnston K**. Balloon angioplasty: predictive factors for long-term success. Semin Vasc Surg. 1989;3:117-22.
12. **Ameli FM, et al**. Predictors of surgical outcome in patients undergoing aortobifemoral bypass reconstruction. J Cardiovasc Surg (Torino). 1990;31:333-9.
13. **Wilson SE, Wolf GL, Cross AP**. Percutaneous transluminal angioplasty versus operation for peripheral arteriosclerosis. Report of a prospective randomized trial in a selected group of patients. J Vasc Surg. 1989;9:1-9.
14. **Holm J, et al**. Chronic lower limb ischaemia. A prospective randomised controlled study comparing the 1-year results of vascular surgery and percutaneous transluminal angioplasty (PTA). Eur J Vasc Surg. 1991;5:517-22.
15. **Sullivan TM, et al**. Percutaneous transluminal angioplasty and primary stenting of the iliac arteries in 288 patients. J Vasc Surg. 1997; 25:829-38; discussion 838-9.
16. **Laborde JC, et al.**, Influence of anatomic distribution of atherosclerosis on the outcome of revascularization with iliac stent placement. J Vasc Interv Radiol. 1995;6:513-21.
17. **Palmaz JC, et al**. Placement of balloon-expandable intraluminal stents in iliac arteries: first 171 procedures. Radiology. 1990;174(3 Pt 2):969-75.
18. **Ponec D, et al**. The Nitinol SMART stent vs Wallstent for suboptimal iliac artery angioplasty: CRISP-US trial results. J Vasc Interv Radiol. 2004;15:911-8.
19. **Palmaz JC, et al**. Stenting of the iliac arteries with the Palmaz stent: experience from a multicenter trial. Cardiovasc Intervent Radiol. 1992;15:291-7.
20. **Henry M, et al**. Palmaz stent placement in iliac and femoropopliteal arteries: primary and secondary patency in 310 patients with 2-4-year follow-up. Radiology. 1995;197:167-74.
21. **Zollikofer CL, Pfyffer M, Redha F, et al**. Arterial stent placement with use of the Wallstent: midterm results of clinical experience. Radiology. 1991;179:449-56.
22. **Vorwerk D, et al**. Aortic and iliac stenoses: follow-up results of stent placement after insufficient balloon angioplasty in 118 cases. Radiology. 1996;198:45-8.
23. **Tetteroo E, et al**. Stent placement after iliac angioplasty: comparison of hemodynamic and angiographic criteria. Dutch Iliac Stent Trial Study Group. Radiology. 1996;201:155-9.
24. **de Vries SO, et al**. Intermittent claudication: cost-effectiveness of revascularization versus exercise therapy. Radiology. 2002;222:25-36.
25. **Hunink MG, et al**. Revascularization for femoropopliteal disease. A decision and cost-effectiveness analysis. JAMA. 1995;274:165-71.
26. **Feinglass J, et al**. Functional status and walking ability after lower extremity bypass grafting or angioplasty for intermittent claudication: results from a prospective outcomes study. J Vasc Surg. 2000;31(1 Pt 1):93-103.
27. **Spronk S, et al**. Intermittent claudication: functional capacity and quality of life after exercise training or percutaneous transluminal angioplasty—systematic review. Radiology. 2005;235:833-42.
28. **Whyman MR, et al**. Randomised controlled trial of percutaneous transluminal angioplasty for intermittent claudication. Eur J Vasc Endovasc Surg. 1996;12:167-72.

29. Jens W, et al. Fate of patients undergoing transluminal angioplasty for lower-limb ischemia. Radiology. 1990;177:559-64.

30. Minar E, et al. Comparison of effects of high-dose and low-dose aspirin on restenosis after femoropopliteal percutaneous transluminal angioplasty. Circulation. 1995;91:2167-73.

31. Clark TW, Groffsky JL, Soulen MC. Predictors of long-term patency after femoropopliteal angioplasty: results from the STAR registry. J Vasc Interv Radiol. 2001;12:923-33.

32. Stokes KR, et al. Five-year results of iliac and femoropopliteal angioplasty in diabetic patients. Radiology. 1990;174(3 Pt 2):977-82.

33. Hewes RC, et al. Long-term results of superficial femoral artery angioplasty. AJR Am J Roentgenol. 1986;146:1025-9.

34. Capek P, McLean GK, Berkowitz HD. Femoropopliteal angioplasty. Factors influencing long-term success. Circulation. 1991;83(2 Suppl): I70-80.

35. Morgenstern, BR, et al. Total occlusions of the femoropopliteal artery: high technical success rate of conventional balloon angioplasty. Radiology. 1989;172(3 Pt 2):937-40.

36. Muradin GS, et al. Balloon dilation and stent implantation for treatment of femoropopliteal arterial disease: meta-analysis. Radiology. 2001;221:137-45.

37. United States Food and Drug Adminstration, Center for Devices and Radiological Health. Intracoil® Self-Expanding Peripheral Stent P000033: Summary of Safety and Effectiveness. 2002.

38. Scheinert D, et al. Prevalence and clinical impact of stent fractures after femoropopliteal stenting. J Am Coll Cardiol. 2005;45:312-5.

39. Vroegindeweij D, et al. Balloon angioplasty combined with primary stenting versus balloon angioplasty alone in femoropopliteal obstructions: A comparative randomized study. Cardiovasc Intervent Radiol. 1997;20:420-5.

40. Schillinger M, et al. Balloon angioplasty versus implantation of nitinol stents in the superficial femoral artery. N Engl J Med. 2006;354:1879-88.

41. Adam DJ, et al. Bypass versus angioplasty in severe ischaemia of the leg (BASIL): multi-centre, randomised controlled trial. Lancet. 2005;366:1925-34.

42. Kudo T, et al. Changing pattern of surgical revascularization for critical limb ischemia over 12 years: endovascular vs. open bypass surgery. J Vasc Surg. 2006;44:304-13.

43. Timaran CH, et al. Predictors for adverse outcome after iliac angioplasty and stenting for limb-threatening ischemia. J Vasc Surg. 2002;36:507-13.

44. Schwarten DE, Cutcliff WB. Arterial occlusive disease below the knee: treatment with percutaneous transluminal angioplasty performed with low-profile catheters and steerable guide wires. Radiology. 1988;169:71-4.

45. Matsi PJ, Suhonen MT, Pirinen AE, Soimakallio S, Chronic critical lower-limb ischemia: prospective trial of angioplasty with 1-36 months of follow-up. Radiology.1993;188:381-7.

46. Dorros G, et al. Below-the-knee angioplasty: tibioperoneal vessels, the acute outcome. Cathet Cardiovasc Diagn. 1990;19:170-8.

47. Dorros G, et al. Tibioperoneal (outflow lesion) angioplasty can be used as primary treatment in 235 patients with critical limb ischemia: five-year follow-up. Circulation. 2001; 104:2057-62.

48. Soder HK, et al. Prospective trial of infrapopliteal artery balloon angioplasty for critical limb ischemia: angiographic and clinical results. J Vasc Interv Radiol. 2000;11:1021-31.

49. Ansel GM, et al. Cutting balloon angioplasty of the popliteal and infrapopliteal vessels for symptomatic limb ischemia. Catheter Cardiovasc Interv. 2004;61:1-4.

50. Rabbi JF, et al. Early results with infrainguinal cutting balloon angioplasty limits distal dissection. Ann Vasc Surg. 2004;18:640-3.

51. Mauri L, et al. Cutting balloon angioplasty for the prevention of restenosis: results of the Cutting Balloon Global Randomized Trial. Am J Cardiol. 2002;90: 1079-83.

52. Conrad MF, et al. Intermediate results of percutaneous endovascular therapy of femoropopliteal occlusive disease: a contemporary series. J Vasc Surg. 2006;44: 762-9.

53. Wildgruber M, et al. Early endothelial and haematological response to cryoplasty compared to balloon angioplasty of the superficial femoral artery - a pilot study. Br J Radiol. 2007.

54. Laird J, et al. Cryoplasty for the treatment of femoropopliteal arterial disease: results of a prospective, multicenter registry. J Vasc Interv Radiol. 2005;16:1067-73.

55. Laird JR, et al. Cryoplasty for the treatment of femoropopliteal arterial disease: extended follow-up results. J Endovasc Ther. 2006;13(Suppl 2):II52-9.

56. Grundfest WS, et al. Pulsed ultraviolet lasers and the potential for safe laser angioplasty. Am J Surg. 1985;150:220-6.

57. Litvack F, et al. Role of laser and thermal ablation devices in the treatment of vascular diseases. Am J Cardiol. 1988;61:81G-86G.

58. Topaz, O., Plaque removal and thrombus dissolution with the photoacoustic energy of pulsed-wave lasers-biotissue interactions and their clinical manifestations. Cardiology. 1996;87:384-91.

59. Laird JR, et al. Limb salvage following laser-assisted angioplasty for critical limb ischemia: results of the LACI multicenter trial. J Endovasc Ther. 2006;13:1-11.

60. Kandzari DE, et al. Procedural and clinical outcomes with catheter-based plaque excision in critical limb ischemia. J Endovasc Ther. 2006;13:12-22.

61. Duda SH, et al. Drug-eluting and bare nitinol stents for the treatment of atherosclerotic lesions in the superficial femoral artery: long-term results from the SIROCCO trial. J Endovasc Ther. 2006;13:701-10.

62. Commeau PP. Barragan, and P.O. Roquebert, Sirolimus for below the knee lesions: mid-term results of SiroBTK study. Catheter Cardiovasc Interv. 2006;68: 793-8.

63. Siablis D, et al. Sirolimus-eluting versus bare stents for bailout after suboptimal infrapopliteal angioplasty for critical limb ischemia: 6-month angiographic results from a nonrandomized prospective single-center study. J Endovasc Ther. 2005;12:685-95.

64. United States Food and Drug Adminstration, Center for Devices and Radiological Health. GORE VIABAHN™ Endoprosthesis - P040037. 2005. Available from: http://www.fda.gov/cdrh/mda/docs/p040037.html.

65. Bray PJ, Robson WJ, Bray AE. Percutaneous treatment of long superficial femoral artery occlusive disease: efficacy of the Hemobahn stent-graft. J Endovasc Ther. 2003;10:619-28.

66. Bosiers M, et al. Will absorbable metal stent technology change our practice? J Cardiovasc Surg (Torino). 2006;47:393-7.

67. Di Mario C, et al. Drug-eluting bioabsorbable magnesium stent. J Interv Cardiol. 2004; 17:391-5.

68. Peeters P, et al. Preliminary results after application of absorbable metal stents in patients with critical limb ischemia. J Endovasc Ther. 2005;12:1-5.

69. Minar E, et al. Endovascular brachytherapy for prophylaxis of restenosis after femoropopliteal angioplasty : results of a prospective randomized study. Circulation. 2000;102:2694-9.

70. Diehm N, et al. Endovascular brachytherapy after femoropopliteal balloon angioplasty fails to show robust clinical benefit over time. J Endovasc Ther. 2005;12:723-30.

71. Wolfram RM, et al. Endovascular brachytherapy: restenosis in de novo versus recurrent lesions of femoropopliteal artery: the Vienna experience. Radiology, 2005;236:338-42.

72. Wolfram RM, et al. Vascular brachytherapy with 192Ir after femoropopliteal stent implantation in high-risk patients: twelve-month follow-up results from the Vienna-5 trial. Radiology. 2005;236:343-51.

73. Therasse E, et al. External beam radiation to prevent restenosis after superficial femoral artery balloon angioplasty. Circulation. 2005;111:3310-5.

74. Rajagopalan S, et al. Regional angiogenesis with vascular endothelial growth factor in peripheral arterial disease: a phase II randomized, double-blind, controlled study of adenoviral delivery of vascular endothelial growth factor 121 in patients with disabling intermittent claudication. Circulation. 2003;108:1933-8.

75. Emmerich J. Current state and perspective on medical treatment of critical leg ischemia: gene and cell therapy. Int J Low Extrem Wounds. 2005;4:234-41.

76. Lederman RJ, et al. Therapeutic angiogenesis with recombinant fibroblast growth factor-2 for intermittent claudication (the TRAFFIC study): a randomised trial. Lancet. 2002;359:2053-8.

77. **Aviles RJ**, Annex BH, Lederman RJ. Testing clinical therapeutic angiogenesis using basic fibroblast growth factor (FGF-2). Br J Pharmacol. 2003;140:637-46.
78. **Roth SM**, Bandyk DF. Duplex imaging of lower extremity bypasses, angioplasties, and stents. Semin Vasc Surg. 1999;12:275-84.
79. **Back MR**, et al. Utility of duplex surveillance following iliac artery angioplasty and primary stenting. J Endovasc Ther. 2001;8:629-37.
80. **Duda SH**, et al. Sirolimus-eluting versus bare nitinol stent for obstructive superficial femoral artery disease: the SIROCCO II trial. J Vasc Interv Radiol. 2005;16:331-8.
81. **Bosch JL**, Hunink MJ. Meta-analysis of the results of percutaneous transluminal angioplasty and stent placement for aortoiliac occlusive disease. Radiology. 1997;204:87-96.
82. **Lazaris AM**, et al. Factors affecting patency of subintimal infrainguinal angioplasty in patients with critical lower limb ischemia. Eur J Vasc Endovasc Surg. 2006;32:668-74.
83. **Lazaris AM**, et al. Clinical outcome of primary infrainguinal subintimal angioplasty in diabetic patients with critical lower limb ischemia. J Endovasc Ther. 2004;11:447-53.
84. **Vraux H, et al.** Subintimal angioplasty of tibial vessel occlusions in the treatment of critical limb ischaemia: mid-term results. Eur J Vasc Endovasc Surg. 2000;20:441-6.
85. **Topaz O.** Rescue excimer laser angioplasty for treatment of critical limb ischemia. Catheter Cardiovasc Interv. 2004;63:13-4.
86. **Boccalandro F, et al.** Wireless laser-assisted angioplasty of the superficial femoral artery in patients with critical limb ischemia who have failed conventional percutaneous revascularization. Catheter Cardiovasc Interv. 2004;63:7-12.
87. **Keeling WB**, et al. Plaque excision with the Silverhawk catheter: early results in patients with claudication or critical limb ischemia. J Vasc Surg. 2007;45:25-31.
88. **Yancey AE**, et al. Peripheral atherectomy in TransAtlantic InterSociety Consensus type C femoropopliteal lesions for limb salvage. J Vasc Surg. 2006;44:503-9.

KEY REFERENCES

Hirsch AT, et al. ACC/AHA 2005 guidelines for the management of patients with peripheral arterial disease (lower extremity, renal, mesenteric, and abdominal aortic): executive summary a collaborative report from the American Association for Vascular Surgery/Society for Vascular Surgery, Society for Cardiovascular Angiography and Interventions, Society for Vascular Medicine and Biology, Society of Interventional Radiology, and the ACC/AHA Task Force on Practice Guidelines (Writing Committee to Develop Guidelines for the Management of Patients With Peripheral Arterial Disease) endorsed by the American Association of Cardiovascular and Pulmonary Rehabilitation; National Heart, Lung, and Blood Institute; Society for Vascular Nursing; TransAtlantic Inter-Society Consensus; and Vascular Disease Foundation. J Am Coll Cardiol. 2006;47:1239-312. *This reference represents the most up to date consensus guidelines for the management of patients with peripheral arterial disease.*

Norgren L, et al. Inter-Society Consensus for the Management of Peripheral Arterial Disease (TASC II). Eur J Vasc Endovasc Surg. 2007;33(Suppl 1):S1-75. *This reference represents the most up to date international consensus guidelines for the management of patients with peripheral arterial disease.*

Scheinert D, et al. Prevalence and clinical impact of stent fractures after femoropopliteal stenting. J Am Coll Cardiol. 2005;45:312-5. *A key reference describing the frequency and outcomes of fem-pop stent fracture.*

Schillinger M, et al. Balloon angioplasty versus implantation of nitinol stents in the superficial femoral artery. N Engl J Med. 2006;354:1879-88. *Landmark randomized controlled trial showing that primary stenting is superior to provisional stenting in fem-pop arteries.*

Adam DJ, et al. Bypass versus angioplasty in severe ischaemia of the leg (BASIL): multicentre, randomised controlled trial. Lancet. 2005;366:1925-34. *Largest randomized trial regarding management of critical limb ischemia patients showing that a strategy of percutaneous intervention first is less expensive than surgery with very similar clinical outcomes.*

Wildgruber M, et al. Early endothelial and haematological response to cryoplasty compared to balloon angioplasty of the superficial femoral artery - a pilot study. Br J Radiol. 2007. *Trial demonstrating that the underlying theoretical benefit of cryoplasty is not valid.*

Duda SH, et al. Drug-eluting and bare nitinol stents for the treatment of atherosclerotic lesions in the superficial femoral artery: long-term results from the SIROCCO trial. J Endovasc Ther. 2006;13:701-10. *Randomized clinical trial demonstrating equivolence of sirolimus-eluting self-expanding nitinol stents to bare metal stents.*

Therasse E, et al. External beam radiation to prevent restenosis after superficial femoral artery balloon angioplasty. Circulation. 2005;111:3310-5. *A promising study showing benefit for external beam radiation for in-stent restenosis in the femoral artery.*

Emmerich J. Current state and perspective on medical treatment of critical leg ischemia: gene and cell therapy. Int J Low Extrem Wounds. 2005;4:234-41. *Best current summary and review of angiogenesis therapies for critical limb ischemia.*

Chapter 7

Surgical Revascularization of Intermittent Claudication and Critical Limb Ischemia

OLIVER AALAMI, MD
JON S. MATSUMURA, MD

1. What is the pre-op evaluation and management of the patient scheduled for surgical revascularization?
2. When should I refer for surgical revascularization of aortoiliac?
3. When should I refer for surgical revascularization of femoral-popliteal?
4. When should I refer for surgical revascularization of tibioperoneal?
5. What are the complications and risks of surgical revascularization?

When To Refer Patients With Intermittent Claudication For Surgical Revascularization

Vascular surgeons have knowledge of the full range of medical, endovascular, and open operative revascularization techniques and risks. Several other specialists, including interventional cardiologists, interventional radiologists, and vascular medicine interventionalists, can provide excellent medical and endovascular skills, and have also become familiar with the indications and risks of open operative revascularization. Any of these physicians are competent to evaluate and treat patients with claudication and critical ischemia. However, some clinicians may favor one approach over others, and it is helpful for the primary care physician to have familiarity with the many options now available to patients with peripheral arterial disease (PAD).

PAD is a common manifestation of atherosclerosis and can present with a broad range of symptoms. The Fontaine classification distinguishes patients based on their symptoms (Table 7-1). Intermittent claudication (IC), Fontaine stage I-II, is one of the most common symptoms of PAD. The word claudication is derived from the Latin word for "limp" (*claudicatio*), but has evolved to describe pain associated with exercise. Symptoms are typically very predictable, with onset at the same level and duration of activity which is often quantified with walking distance (e.g., two blocks). Claudication symptoms due to arterial disease resolve with standing and rest and do not require laying flat. The location of muscle cramping or pain should correlate with the location of arterial disease. Most commonly, femoral artery blockage causes calf cramping, aching, or weakness. If the external iliac, common femoral, or profunda femoral are affected, the pain may also occur in the thigh. Patients with aortic, common iliac, or hypogastric artery disease will also have buttock muscle pain and men may have erectile dysfunction.

Medical management, as outlined in Chapter 5, is the mainstay of treatment for patients with intermittent claudication. Referral to a vascular specialist is recommended to confirm the diagnosis and emphasize exercise and risk factor modification. Vascular specialists recognize rare arterial conditions, such as cystic adventitial disease, popliteal entrapment, and popliteal aneurysms that may masquerade as classic atherosclerosis, and require different therapeutic approaches. The vascular specialist should inform the patient of all therapeutic options relative to the patient's disability and extent of vascular disease and follow up for possible progression of disease. This discussion of risks (detailed later in this chapter) and limited durability of endovascular and open procedures helps educate the patient about the importance of risk factor modification and the relative safety of exercise programs. If the disease progresses to interfere with the patient's lifestyle or work demands, then endovascular or operative revascularization may be considered. On the other hand, if the patient leads a sedentary lifestyle or has advanced cardiac, pulmonary, or musculoskeletal disease that is the primary limitation of activity, then revascularization is not recommended.

Table 7-1. Fontaine Classification For Lower-Extremity Arterial Occlusive Disease*

Fontaine Classification	Patient Presentation
I	Asymptomatic
II	Claudication
III	Ischemic rest pain
IV	Ischemic ulceration/necrosis

*Fontaine R, Kim M, Kieny R. Die chirurgische Behandlung der peripheren Durch-blutungsstoerungen. Helv Chir Acta. 1954;5/6:199-533.

When the decision for intervention is being considered, the risks and benefits must be carefully weighed. This risk/benefit analysis must take into account several factors: 1) disability caused by the symptoms, 2) location and characteristics of the lesion, 3) individualized risk of the considered intervention, and 4) predicted survival of the patient. The following are examples of each of these: generally, intervention for intermittent claudication should only be performed when the disability significantly limits a patient's lifestyle. Anatomic location and characteristics predict long-term patency; for example, iliac stenoses have a high success rate with endovascular treatment and relative high durability compared to long segment femoral occlusion with distal calf vessel disease. A patient with a hypercoagulable disorder may be a poor candidate for any type of intervention for claudication. Patients with untreatable malignancy, advanced heart failure, and severe dementia are rarely candidates for revascularization for claudication. Vascular specialists should be expert at evaluating and synthesizing these individualized risk assessments. Over treatment may occur if technical feasibility is the only consideration.

When To Refer Patients With Critical Limb Ischemia For Surgical Revascularization

Critical limb ischemia (CLI) is the progression of arterial occlusive disease to stage III or IV infrainguinal arteriosclerosis, where patients present with rest pain, ischemic ulceration, or gangrene. The definition of CLI by the Trans-Atlantic Inter-Society Consensus (TASC) conference is: 1) persistent, recurring ischemic rest pain requiring opiate analgesia for at least 2 weeks, 2) ulceration or gangrene of the foot or toes, and 3) ankle systolic pressure less than 50 mmHg or toe systolic pressure less than 30 mmHg. Unfortunately, it is difficult to predict which patients with claudication will progress through the Fontaine stages to CLI. Up to 50% of patients are asymptomatic 6 months prior to their amputations for CLI. Increasing age and smoking are major risk factors, but diabetes remains the greatest risk factor. Amputations are 10 times more frequent in diabetic patients with PAD, such that up to 45% of all major amputees are diabetic. Prompt referral to a vascular surgeon is advised, as time-to-treatment may be an important component to limb salvage. In sharp contrast to claudication symptoms alone, patients with CLI undergo revascularization unless they are not ambulatory, no standard risk options are available, or the patient is terminally ill (predicted survival less than a few months).

CLI can be divided into acute and chronic limb ischemia. Ischemic symptoms of 14 days duration or less is classified as acute limb ischemia. These patients typically have not developed adequate collateralization and are at increased risk for limb loss. Chronic ischemia patients typically have well-developed collaterals and report gradual worsening of symptoms over

Table 7-2.   Rutherford Criteria of Acute Limb Ischemia*

Class 1	Viable limb even without therapeutic intervention
Class 2a	Threatened limb not requiring immediate revascularization (intact motor and sensory function)
Class 2b	Threatened limb requiring immediate revascularization (compromised muscle function or sensory symptoms)
Class 3	Irreversibly ischemic limb that is unsalvageable

*Suggested standards for reports dealing with lower extremity ischemia. Prepared by the Ad Hoc Committee on Reporting Standards, Society for Vascular Surgery/North American Chapter, International Society for Cardiovascular Surgery. J Vasc Surg. 1986;4:80-94.

time. Acute limb ischemia is classified using the Rutherford criteria (Table 7-2). A Class 1 limb is viable and does not require immediate therapeutic intervention. Class 2a limbs are not immediately threatened but do require therapeutic intervention. These patients have intact motor and sensory function. Class 2b limbs are immediately threatened and require urgent revascularization for salvage: patients with compromised muscle function or acute neurological symptoms should be referred to the emergency room. Class 3 limbs are irreversibly ischemic with tissue infarction where functional limb salvage is not possible.

By definition, most patients with chronic CLI (rest pain, ischemic ulcer, and gangrene) will have limb-loss unless revascularization is accomplished. However, even these patients have a broad spectrum of clinical presentation and outcome. In some patients with chronic lower-extremity ischemia, Taylor and Porter reported successful preservation of limb viability using general supportive measures alone in up to 25% to 40% of cases (1). In other patients with poor overall prognosis, high operative risk, and who are not ambulatory immediately prior to the onset of their disease, revascularization is not attempted. Occasionally, this includes patients who have had previous amputation, have no functional use of the limb, and develop ischemia of their stump. Some patients have undergone multiple previous procedures with progressively diminishing patency intervals of months or weeks, and futility must be recognized. Those not deemed candidates for revascularization are evaluated for the appropriate level of amputation to relieve their symptoms and prevent systemic manifestations. Occasionally, hospice care must be considered instead of amputation. These complex types of scenarios require seasoned judgment, restraint from the usual aggressive limb-salvage strategy, and caring communication with patient and family.

Revascularization Options and Outcomes

Patients with symptoms of rest pain, ischemic ulceration, or gangrene require prompt referral to a vascular surgeon. Treatment of patients with CLI who are candidates for revascularization may be via open surgical or en-dovascular approach depending on the location and characteristics of the patient's atherosclerotic disease, availability of autogenous conduit when infrainguinal revascularization is needed, and overall medical condition.

Aortoiliac disease limited to the iliac vessels may be treated with balloon angioplasty and provisional stenting in patients with focal stenotic lesions. Three-year patency rates range between 74% and 86% (2). Severe occlusive disease involving the distal aorta and its bifurcation may be treated with aor-toiliac endarterectomy. Long complete occlusions often require an open by-pass procedure, such as an aortobifemoral bypass (Figure 7-1a). Perioperative mortality in patients who are appropriately risk-stratified is less than 3%. Graft occlusion is the most common late complication of these procedures. Brewster et al reported a 5% to 10% 5-year incidence of occlusion in the first 5 years and a 15% to 30% incidence after 10 years. For patients with severe comorbid disease, alternative open operations are available that do not re-quire laparotomy or aortic clamping. Axillo-femoral bypass combined with a femoro-femoral bypass is the most common extra-anatomic bypass used for aorto-iliac occlusive disease in such patients, as it avoids the metabolic, renal, and cardiac stress associated with aortic cross-clamping (see Figures 7-1b, 7-1c). Reports of 5-year primary patency rates have ranged between 39% and 85%, although a recent report from 1996 reports equivalent 5-year primary pa-tency rates between aorto-femoral bypass and axillo-femoral bypass (80% vs. 74%, respectively) using modern techniques of externally supported grafts, careful tunneling, and medial proximal anastomosis. For patients who can tol-erate a thoracotomy, the thoraco-femoral bypass is a durable alternative by-pass procedure. Favorable 4-year primary patency rates are 86% with secondary patency rates approaching 100% (3). This operation is usually re-served for patients with previous failed abdominal aortic operations. Long-term survival of patients with CLI is relatively poor. Thirty percent of patients will not survive beyond 5 years; 60% will not survive beyond 10 years.

Femoral-popliteal disease most often involves the superficial femoral ar-tery (SFA). Interestingly, a patent deep femoral artery provides sufficient flow to the lower extremity through collaterals in 80% of patients. Infrainguinal bypass graft patencies are superior when a vein graft is used, particularly when the vein graft is at least 3 mm in diameter. Above-knee vein bypass grafts have a 76% 5-year patency rate, while polyester or poly-tetrafluorethylene (PTFE) grafts have a 52% 5-year patency rate. Four-year below-knee PTFE graft patency ranges between 12% and 54%, while vein grafts in this position have patency rates between 49% and 76% (4). Minimal differences in patency rates are noted between in-situ and reversed vein conduits. Poor runoff is a predictor of poor graft patency rates. Modified PTFE grafts, such as tapered, hooded, carbon-coated or heparin-bonded PTFE grafts, have been designed to improve on graft patency. Walluscheck et al reported 1- and 2-year primary patency rates for below-knee bypasses with heparin-bonded PTFE in a series of 40 patients to be

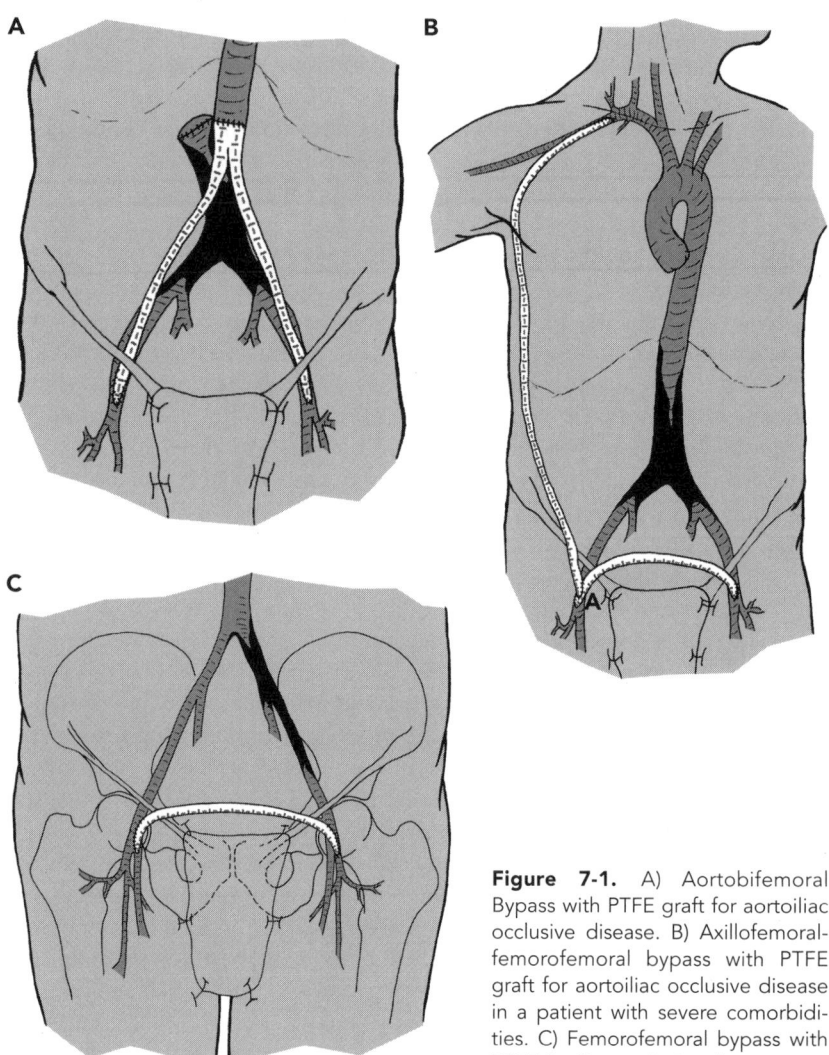

Figure 7-1. A) Aortobifemoral Bypass with PTFE graft for aortoiliac occlusive disease. B) Axillofemoral-femorofemoral bypass with PTFE graft for aortoiliac occlusive disease in a patient with severe comorbidities. C) Femorofemoral bypass with PTFE for iliac occlusive disease.

92% and 81%, respectively. Prospective long-term results and randomized trials are not available.

Endovascular approaches to infrainguinal lesions are being used more widely. These procedures include angioplasty and selective stenting, subintimal angioplasty to cross total occlusions, and fibrinolysis of acutely thrombosed vessels/grafts. Lower initial morbidity and mortality rates compared to infrainguinal bypasses are being reported (3% and 0% vs. 10% and 3%) (5). When compared to bypass procedures, in the BASIL trial, angioplasty was favored in the first year. If the patient's life expectancy is greater than

2 years, then open bypass procedures may have superior patency rates with fewer reinterventions (6). The advent of nitinol self-expanding stents may improve the results of angioplasty. Previous randomized trials with balloon-expandable stents did not show superior results, but, recently, 12-month restenosis rates of the SFA have been shown to be lower in patients who received primary self-expanding nitinol stents compared to patients who received angioplasty and selective stenting. Conrad et al also recently demonstrated equivalent 24-month secondary patency and limb-salvage rates with femoropopliteal PTA/stenting between TASC A/B patients and the more extensively diseased TASC C/D patients (5) (Table 7-3). Dosluoglu et al report higher limb-salvage rates in their series of patients with CLI who

Table 7-3.   TransAtlantic Inter-Society Consensus (TASC) Classification of Aortoiliac Lesions and Treatment Recommendations*

TASC	Description	Treatment Recommendation
A	• Unilateral or bilateral stenosis of CIA • Unilateral or bilateral single short (<3cm) stenosis of EIA	Endovascular
B	• Short stenosis of infrarenal aorta • Unilateral CIA occlusion • Single or multiple stenosis totaling 3-10 cm involving the EIA (not extending into the CFA) • Unilateral EIA occlusion not involving the origin of internal iliac or CFA	Endovascular preferred
C	• Bilateral CIA occlusions • Bilateral EIA stenosis 3-10 cm long not extending into the CFA • Unilateral EIA stenosis extending into the CFA • Unilateral EIA occlusion that involves the origins of the internal iliac and/or CFA • Heavy calcified unilateral EIA occlusion with or without involvement of origins of internal iliac and/or CFA	Surgery preferred (if good-risk patient)
D	• Infra-renal aortoiliac occlusion • Diffuse disease involving the aorta and both iliac arteries requiring treatment • Diffuse multiple stenoses involving the unilateral CIA, EIA and CFA • Unilateral occlusions of both CIA and EIA • Bilateral occlusions of the EIA • Iliac stenoses in patients with AAA requiring treatment and not amenable to endograft placement or other lesions requiring open aortic or iliac surgery	Surgery

*Norgren L, Hiatt WR, Dormandy JA, et al on behalf of the TASC II Working Group. Inter-Society Consensus for the Management of Peripheral Arterial Disease (TASC II). J Vasc Surg. 2007;45(1 Suppl):S5-S67.

had preferential endovascular therapy (7). These data support the use of PTA and selective stenting as a primary therapy for patients with femoropopliteal occlusive disease, and open bypass procedures for endovascular failures.

Diabetic patients often have tibioperoneal disease requiring a distal bypass below the knee or even to the arteries in the foot (Figure 7-2). Special attention must be paid to ensure adequate inflow as well as outflow prior to embarking on distal revascularization. Vein grafts have superior patency rates in this position as in other positions. Five-year actuarial, primary, and secondary patency rates of dorsalis pedis bypass grafts with vein as conduit has been reported to be 68%, 82%, and 87%, respectively. Patient survival rate over this period was 57% (8). Intraoperative modification of vein by-

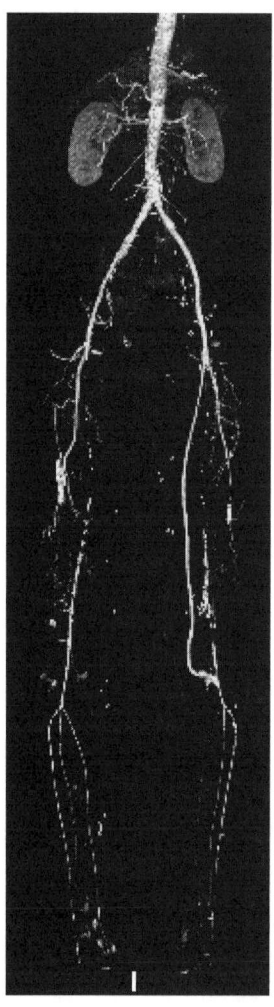

Figure 7-2. CT Angiogram of femoropopliteal bypass graft

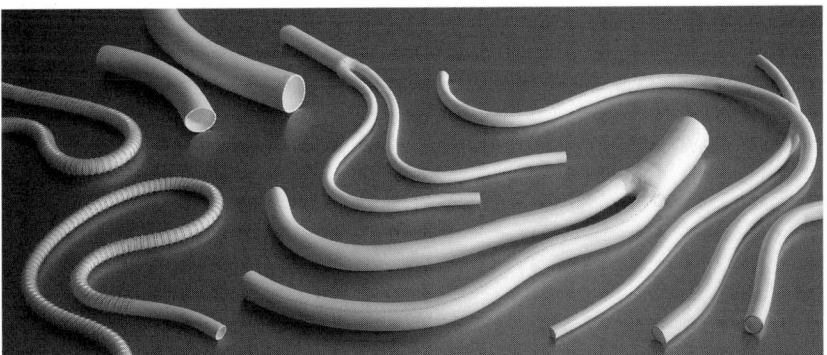

Figure 7-3. Image of polytetrafluoroethylene (PTFE) grafts (Image courtesy of W. L. Gore & Associates, Inc.)

pass grafts using a molecular transcription factor E2F decoy to prevent neointimal hyperplasia did not show improved primary patency rates compared to control vein conduits. When insufficient vein is available, either a composite graft or a synthetic graft (e.g., PTFE) may be used (Figure 7-3). Creation of a distal anastomotic vein-cuff to decrease the compliance mismatch between the graft and the target artery has been shown to improve patency rates of distal bypass procedures. Two-year below-knee bypass patencies were improved from 29% to 52% when a vein cuff was added to PTFE bypass grafts. Limb salvage was also improved from 62% to 84%. Bypass graft patency rates vary depending on location as well as the conduit used (Table 7-4).

For patients with tissue loss, early referral to a vascular surgeon allows for careful planning of preoperative work-up, sequence, and urgency of revascularization that will optimize overall patency and functional limb salvage. Generally, bypass is favored when there is a good autogenous vein, long segment occlusion, and an adequate target. However, the vascular surgeon must evaluate many other contributing factors, such as previous

Table 7-4.   Bypass Graft Patency Rates

Bypass Procedure	4-yr Primary Patency Rate	5-yr Primary Patency Rate
Aortobifemoral bypass	—	80%
Axillofemoral bypass	—	74%
Fem-pop above-knee (vein)	—	76%
Fem-op bove-knee (PTFE)	—	52%
Fem-pop below-knee (vein)	49%-76%	—
Fem-pop below-knee (PTFE)	12%-54%	—
Dorsalis pedis bypass (vein)	—	68%

operations, contractures, overlying skin health, amount and location of tissue loss, and alternative wound etiologies such as venous stasis, neurotrophic conditions, and decubitus ulcers. Often, staged procedures are necessary with initial drainage of infection, then revascularization, followed by wound closure/management procedures such as skin grafts and toe amputation.

Complications of Revascularization

Many complications affecting multiple organ systems may occur following arterial revascularization. They can be categorized as systemic, graft-related, and wound problems. Incidences vary depending on the extent of the procedures, but systemic problems are dominated by cardiac, pulmonary, and renal complications. Graft-related complications include occlusions, infections, and anastomotic aneurysms. Wound complications most often are hemorrhage, skin necrosis, localized infection, or lymphatic leak. Vascular surgeons, primary care physicians, nurses, and other specialists expend a significant amount of time in the care of patients before and after operative bypass because of these systemic, graft, and wound complications. More importantly, the burden of these complications on functional patient recovery weigh heavily in the decision-making process.

Due to the high prevalence of cardiac disease in patients with PAD, coronary complications remain a major cause of morbidity and are the leading cause of death following revascularization. In the last decade, the rates of peri-operative myocardial infarction have ranged between 0% and 7% in patients undergoing open abdominal aortic surgery. Slightly higher rates between 1.6% and 14% were reported for patients undergoing infrainguinal bypass procedures. These rates reflect high-risk cohorts, and routine preoperative screening has been suggested. Although preoperative coronary revascularization failed to reduce short- or long-term mortality after major peripheral vascular operation in the Veterans Affairs randomized trial, some randomized trials have shown reduction of coronary events with the routine use of perioperative beta blockade and routine active patient warming (8). Most clinicians also use postopearative antiplatelet agents and perioperative statin therapy.

Patients undergoing upper abdominal or thoracic procedures and those with a history of smoking are at increased risk for the development of respiratory complications in vascular surgery. Common manifestations of postoperative respiratory problems include atelectasis, bronchospasm, aspiration, bronchitis, and pneumonia. The latter is a major complication; the Centers for Disease Control reported in 1994 the mortality rates from nosocomial pneumonia to range between 20% and 50%. Risk factors include emphysema, asthma, smoking history, and obesity. Maneuvers to help minimize complications include preopearative optimization of pulmonary function, early extubation with aggressive pulmonary toilet, and early ambulation to help prevent atelectasis and bronchopneumonia.

Renal failure due to acute tubular necrosis is the most common manifestation of renal complications in the vascular patient. The etiology is most often due to ischemic injury secondary to shock, intra-operative clamping, atheroembolism, or toxic injury. Adequate hydration of patients scheduled to receive intravenous contrast is important. Many centers have adopted protocols with the administration of sodium bicarbonate or the anti-oxidant N-acetylcysteine for renal protection based on small randomized trials. The use of mannitol before aortic clamping and renal dose dopamine infusions have been used to help minimize the incidence of oliguric uremia after aortic operation.

Early graft thrombosis is most often due to technical factors and is usually addressed immediately with thrombectomy and bypass revision. If no technical problems are identified, empiric anticoagulation is initiated and a hypercoagulable work-up may be pursued. Graft thrombosis during the first 2 years most often represents new intimal hyperplasia within the graft or at either anastomosis. Later graft failure often occurs due to native vessel disease progression. Thrombolysis or thrombectomy may be performed for graft occlusion with follow-up arteriography to uncover the underlying lesion to guide subsequent endovascular treatment or revision. Randomized trials showed comparable outcomes with either strategy, although subset analysis suggests that tailoring therapy may help in some patient subgroups. For example, the surgery versus thrombolysis for ischemia of the lower extremity trial (STILE) showed decreased planned surgical procedures, higher limb-salvage rates and shorter hospital stays for the subgroup of patients who underwent thrombolysis of either native arterial bypasses or bypass grafts less than 14 days after presenting with acute ischemia (10).

The most devastating graft-related complication is a graft infection. It most often requires complete removal of the entire conduit with revascularization through un-infected tissue. The incidence has been reported as between 1% and 5%. Most graft infections occur in the groin and present with cellulitis, persistent drainage, anastomotic pseudoaneurysm, or bleeding. More than 50% of cases are *Staphylococcus epidermidis* infections, but methicillin-resistant *Staphylococcus aureus,* as well as more virulent gram-negative infections are on the rise. Often, extra-anatomic bypasses with autogenous vein must be performed in order to stay out of infected tissue plains. Some centers use rifampin-soaked prosthetic grafts, antibiotic-eluting beads, or cadaveric arterial homografts with tissue flaps in infected fields when autogenous vein is not available.

Anastomotic aneurysms are late complications that are typically due to native arterial degeneration, suture disruption, graft deterioration, mechanical stress or infection. Small, asymptomatic anastomotic aneurysms are usually observed with serial imaging. Large or symptomatic anastomotic aneurysms require repair due to their risk of rupture.

Aortic surgery carries risk for the rare but unusual complications of aortoenteric fistulae and erectile or ejaculatory dysfunction. The incidence of aortoenteric fistula is less than 1%, but they have a dramatic presentation. They most commonly occur in the distal duodenum. Erosion of the graft through the bowel wall with ensuing infection is thought to be the cause of aortoenteric fistula formation and may be prevented by interposition of retroperitoneal fat or omentum over the graft. Enteric fistulae often present with an upper gastrointestinal "herald bleed" and are diagnosed on upper endoscopy to the distal duodenum or CT scan. Graft removal with extraanatomic bypass is the standard treatment.

Erectile dysfunction may result from interruption of flow to the internal iliac arteries. Ejaculatory dysfunction may manifest itself as retrograde ejaculation if para-aortic autonomic nerve fibers are disrupted.

Pre-Operative Evaluation and Management

The high incidence of coronary artery disease in patients undergoing arterial revascularization was highlighted by Hertzer in 1984. The American College of Cardiology (ACC) and the American Heart Association (AHA) developed guidelines for perioperative cardiovascular evaluation for noncardiac surgery in 2002. Patients are clinically stratified to high, intermediate, or low coronary risk. High-risk patients are evaluated and treated aggressively before surgery as they typically have unstable coronary artery disease. The low-risk patients do not usually require noninvasive stress imaging pre-operatively. The intermediate group should be further evaluated with noninvasive stress testing. However, the approach to revascularization of those with reversible coronary artery ischemia is unclear, as McFalls et al reported in the CARP trial (Coronary Artery Revascularization Prophylaxis) that preoperative coronary artery revascularization does not improve perioperative or long-term survival after elective vascular surgery, including aortic procedures and lower-extremity bypass. Two small randomized trials suggest that perioperative beta blockade improves patient outcomes, although larger confirmatory trials are underway. Until then, perioperative beta blockers should be strongly considered in patients without contraindications with a goal heart rate below 60 beats-per-minute.

Fundamentals of medical therapy, although obvious, should not be overlooked. Smoking cessation is universally recommended as early as possible before and after the planned procedure because it reduces systemic, graft, and wound complications and improves long-term outcomes. Strict blood glucose control has become standard for all perioperative patients with liberal use of insulin drips in the intensive care unit. Antihypertensive treatment, statins, and antiplatelet therapy are also routine if not contraindicated.

Conclusion

Peripheral arterial disease is a marker for systemic vascular disease and is associated with increased morbidity and mortality. Intermittent claudication itself has a relatively benign natural history. Medical management is appropriate until patients experience lifestyle-limiting disability. In contrast, progression to rest pain, non-healing wounds, or limb-threatening ischemia are standard indications for vascular intervention in ambulatory patients. Early referral of patients to a vascular specialist allows for timely and appropriate intervention in the context of global team management of these often complex and challenging patient problems.

REFERENCES

1. Taylor LM Jr., Porter JM. Clinical and anatomic considerations for surgery in femoropopliteal disease and the results of surgery. Circulation. 1991;83(2 Suppl):I63-9.
2. Klein WM, van der Graaf Y, Seegers J, et al. Dutch iliac stent trial: long-term results in patients randomized for primary or selective stent placement. Radiology. 2006;238:734-44.
3. McCarthy WJ, Mesh CL, McMillan WD, et al. Descending thoracic aorta-to-femoral artery bypass: ten years' experience with a durable procedure. J Vasc Surg. 1993;17:336-47; discussion 47-8.
4. Veith FJ, Gupta SK, Ascer E, et al. Six-year prospective multicenter randomized comparison of autologous saphenous vein and expanded polytetrafluoroethylene grafts in infrainguinal arterial reconstructions. J Vasc Surg. 1986;3:104-14.
5. Conrad MF, Cambria RP, Stone DH, et al. Intermediate results of percutaneous endovascular therapy of femoropopliteal occlusive disease: a contemporary series. J Vasc Surg. 2006;44:762-9.
6. Adam DJ, Beard JD, Cleveland T, et al. Bypass versus angioplasty in severe ischaemia of the leg (BASIL): multicentre, randomised controlled trial. Lancet. 2005;366:1925-34.
7. Dosluoglu HH, O'Brien-Irr MS, Lukan J, et al. Does preferential use of endovascular interventions by vascular surgeons improve limb salvage, control of symptoms, and survival of patients with critical limb ischemia? Am J Surg. 2006;192:572-6.
8. Pomposelli FB Jr., Marcaccio EJ, Gibbons GW, et al. Dorsalis pedis arterial bypass: durable limb salvage for foot ischemia in patients with diabetes mellitus. J Vasc Surg. 1995;21:375-84.
9. McFalls EO, Ward HB, Moritz TE, et al. Coronary-artery revascularization before elective major vascular surgery. N Engl J Med. 2004;351:2795-804.
10. Results of a prospective randomized trial evaluating surgery versus thrombolysis for ischemia of the lower extremity. The STILE trial. Ann Surg. 1994;220:251-66; discussion 66-8.

KEY REFERENCES

Klein WM, van der Graaf Y, Seegers J, et al. Dutch iliac stent trial: long-term results in patients randomized for primary or selective stent placement. Radiology. 2006;238:734-44.

279 patients with iliac disease were randomized to receive primary stents or percutaneous transluminal angioplasty with selective stent placement for mean pressure gradient >10 mmHg. This study reported greater than 80% 5-year patency rates with both selective and primary iliac artery stenting. Patients treated with PTA and selective stent placement in iliac artery had a better outcome for symptomatic success (improvement in Fontaine classification by one grade), but there was no difference in iliac patency, ABIs or quality of life between the two groups.

McFalls EO, Ward HB, Moritz TE, et al. Coronary-artery revascularization before elective major vascular surgery. N Engl J Med. 2004;351:2795-804. *Patients with significant coronary artery disease (but not left main coronary disease, aortic stenosis, or poor left ventricular function) requiring lower-extremity bypass or aortic operation can undergo vascular surgery with low morbidity and mortality, and these results cannot be improved by coronary artery revascularization before vascular surgery. Late mortality was also not improved by coronary revascularization. This randomized trial challenges the common assumption that routine aggressive cardiac testing and revascularization is indicated for all patients having major vascular operations.*

Adam DJ, Beard JD, Cleveland T, et al. BASIL TRIAL. Lancet. 2005;366:1925-34. *When comparing surgery-first to angioplasty-first for patients with rest pain, ulceration, or gangrene of the leg, no significant difference in amputation-free survival or mortality was noted at 2 years. In post hoc analysis, there was a trend towards greater amputation-free survival at 5 years for surgery-first patients.*

Results of a prospective randomized trial evaluating surgery versus thrombolysis for ischemia of the lower extremity. The STILE trial. Ann Surg. 1994;220:251-66; discussion 66-8. *Patients with acute lower-extremity ischemia deterioration of <14 days had lower amputation rates and lower hospital stay days when treated with thrombolysis rather than open surgical intervention. Surgical therapy was superior when patients had lower-extremity ischemia duration >14 days.*

Taylor L, Porter JM. Clinical and anatomic considerations for surgery in femoropopliteal disease and the results of surgery. Circulation. 1991;83(2 Suppl):I63-9. *Overall primary graft patency for all femoropopliteal bypass grafts was 79% at 5-years in this study of 288 operations. Good guality saphenous vein graft had a primary 5-year patency rate of 85% while non-saphenous vein grafts had a 5-year patency rate of 73%.*

Veith FJ, Gupta SK, Ascer E, et al. Six-year prospective multicenter randomized comparison of autologous saphenous vein and expanded polytetrafluoroethylene grafts in infrainguinal arterial reconstructions. J Vasc Surg. 1986;3:104-14. *Every effort should be made to use autologous saphenous vein (ASV) grafts for below-knee bypass grafts. PTFE may be used preferentially in selected poor-risk patients for femoropopliteal bypasses above the knee. No statistically significant difference was noted in 4-year patency between ASV grafts and PTFE grafts, which were in the above-knee popliteal position. Below-knee femoropopliteal 4-year patency rates were 76% for ASV grafts versus 54% for PTFE grafts. Infrapopliteal bypass patency rates were 49% for ASV grafts and only 12% for PTFE grafts.*

Dosluoglu HH, O'Brien-Irr MS, Lukan J, et al. Does preferential use of endovascular interventions by vascular surgeons improve limb salvage, control of symptoms, and survival of patients with critical limb ischemia? Am J Surg. 2006;192:572-6. *A restrospective review of patients who presented with critical limb ischemia showed lower primary amputation rates, improved limb salvage, and shorter length of stay in patients who were preferentially treated with endovascular interventions.*

McCarthy WJ, Mesh CL, McMillan WD, et al. Descending thoracic aorta-to-femoral artery bypass: ten years' experience with a durable procedure. J Vasc Surg. 1993;17:336-47; discussion 347-8. *Descending thoracic aorta-to-femoral artery bypass grafting is safe and extremely durable (100% 4-year patency). It is an excellent reconstruction for survivors of aortic graft infection, those who have had multiple failures of aortic grafts, and patients for whom abdominal exploration would be hazardous.*

Pomposelli FB Jr., Marcaccio EJ, Gibbons GW, et al. Dorsalis pedis arterial bypass: durable limb salvage for foot ischemia in patients with diabetes mellitus. J Vasc Surg. 1995;21:375-84. *A review of 367 consecutive patients undergoing 384 bypass grafts to the dorsalis pedis artery for limb salvage showed actuarial primary patency, secondary patency, and limb salvage rates to be 68%, 82%, and 87%, respectively at 5 years.*

Conrad MF, Cambria RP, Stone DH, et al. Intermediate results of percutaneous endovascular therapy of femoropopliteal occlusive disease: a contemporary series. J Vasc Surg. 2006;44:762-9 *Femoropopliteal angioplasty is associated with low morbidity and mortality. Its success is directly proportional to the burden of disease in the treated vessel. Secondary interventions are often necessary to maintain vessel patency of high- grade lesions. Primary use of endovascular approaches for high- and low-grade lesions in patients with critical limb ischemia is appropriate.*

Chapter 8

Future of Peripheral Arterial Disease Therapy: Angiogenesis and Cell Therapy

EMILE R. MOHLER III, MD

1. What is angiogenesis and how does it work?
2. Are pro-angiogenic cytokines useful for claudication?
3. Are stem cells useful for claudication?
4. What are the risks of angiogenesis?
5. When should I consider a patient for an angiogenesis trial?

Treatment for claudication due to peripheral arterial disease (PAD) includes supervised exercise rehabilitation and prescription of either cilostazol or pentoxyphylline. Despite this therapeutic approach, patients commonly continue to have lifestyle-limiting claudication symptoms. Lower-limb revascularization, especially involving the infrainguinal region, may be achieved with percutaneous or surgical intervention, but this is generally reserved for patients with critical limb ischemia (1). Some patients generate collaterals either spontaneously or in response to exercise-induced ischemia. The evolving understanding of the angiogenic process has led to the concept of therapeutic angiogenesis, whereby pro-angiogenic cytokines and/or cell-based therapy are being tested so as to improve claudication symptoms. This chapter focuses on cytokine and cell-based strategies under development to treat claudication symptoms.

Angiogenesis

The development of a vascular network in the embryo involves the in situ differentiation of primitive angioblasts to endothelial cells, a process called vasculogenesis (2). As the embryo grows, the further development of a vascular network depends on angiogenesis, a distinct mechanism of vascular growth in which the blood vessels expand via division of existing cells within the vascular network. Until recently, the sole mechanism for development of new vascular networks in response to ischemia was thought to be due to angiogenesis. The angiogenic response involves vascular sprouting and intucesseption, followed by myogenesis (3). However, recent evidence indicates that the adult bone marrow is a source of cells that can participate in post-natal vasculogenesis. Evidence for this theory came from Asahara and colleagues, who found that peripheral blood contains cells that differentiate into endothelial cells (4). They demonstrated that these endothelial progenitor cells (EPCs) incorporate into sites of active angiogenesis in an animal model. These are thought to participate in vascular homeostasis, ischemic vasculogenesis, and tumor angiogenesis.

Despite recent advances in understanding vascular homeostasis and angiogenesis, there remain many unanswered questions, and the process is still not completely understood. An area of controversy is the phenotypic characterization of EPCs. These cells are thought to be mobilized from the bone marrow and circulate in the blood stream in response to various stimuli, such as pro-angiogenic cytokines (Figure 8-1). However, also circulating in the blood stream are mature endothelial cells that either are apparently sloughed off from the endothelium or perhaps have matured, but have not been incorporated into the endothelial lining. These cells, termed circulating endothelial cells (CECs), have some similar surface markers found in progenitor endothelial cells. Some studies used only one or two cell surface markers to distinguish EPCs from mature cells and thus may not represent a pure population of EPCs. In addition, there are EPCs that seem to be derived from the myeloid cell line and therefore of macrophage lineage. The CECs are, however, distinguished from EPCs due to their reduced ability to participate in post-natal vasculogenesis. Scientists have also identified highly proliferative endothelial cells embedded in the lining of blood vessels (5). These cells may be resident from embryonic development or are perhaps derived from adult circulating progenitor cells.

Various animal models have been used to investigate the role of bone-marrow-derived EPCs in the vasculogenic process. Some of these studies involve bone marrow transplantation using enhanced green fluorescent protein (GFP) to follow the fate of the EPC and indicate that the precursor cells incorporate into capillaries in the ischemic hind limbs. One study showed that ex-vivo expanded human EPCs transplanted into a nude mice with hindlimb ischemia improved blood flow and capillary density (4). There is also evidence to suggest that occlusion of a major artery results in expansion of native collateral arteries to restore blood flow. This arteriogenesis is thought to occur due to outward remodeling of pre-existing intra-arterial connections. Monocytes/macrophages are reported to accumulate around growing collateral vessels and speculated to provide a nu-

Mechanism of Progenitor Cell Mobilization

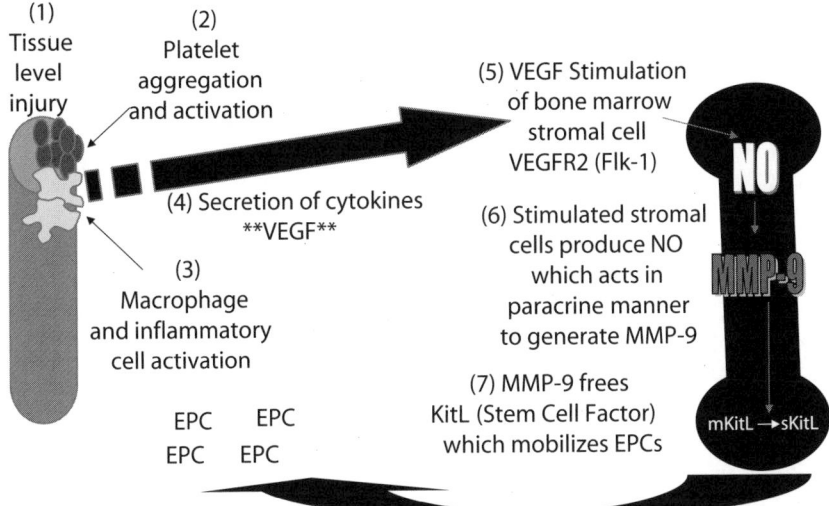

Figure 8-1.   Schematic showing EPC release from bone marrow. Proangiogenic cytokines such as vascular endothelial growth factor (VEGF) are generated from endothelial cells in response to tissue ischemia. The VEGF receptor is then activated and stimulates nitric oxide synthase production and nitric oxide generation which acts in a paracrine fashion to stimulate production of matrix metalloproteinase 9 (MMP-9). Lit ligand (also known as stem cell factor) is freed by MMP-9 and this facilitates EPC mobilization into the circulation.

trient role, including release growth factors, cytokines, and various proteases. Thus, the angiogenic response appears to involve cellular processes beyond EPCs to facilitate rapid reperfusion.

Clinical studies indicate that EPCs are a biomarker of atherosclerotic disease progression; studies show an inverse correlation between cardiovascular mortality and EPC level. Cardiovascular risk factors such as hypercholesterolemia, hypertension, and diabetes mellitus, as well as advanced age, negatively affect the circulating EPC number (6,7). However, drugs such as HMG-Co A reductase inhibitors (statins) and erythropoietin, and exercise, mobilize EPCs from the bone marrow into the circulation. One study showed that while baseline levels of EPCs and ECs were similar among all subjects, young healthy subjects demonstrated significantly greater levels of progenitor cells (cell positive for the surface markers CD34 and 133) than older healthy and PAD subjects (8). Levels of EPCs and ECs tended to increase in all subjects after exercise; however, increases in progenitor cells were only observed in young healthy and PAD subjects. Further, trends in the magnitude of change of subsets with exercise were most similar between young and PAD subjects. These findings suggest that aging may reduce baseline circulating levels of progenitor cells, but not EPCs or ECs, and that exercise-induced mobilization of subsets may differ depending on age and presence of PAD.

Pro-Angiogenic Cytokines and Claudication

There are two key processes that determine the amount of blood flow to skeletal muscle in patients with PAD. The first is the degree of arterial occlusion and the second is the degree to which an endogenous arteriogenic response is mounted to compensate for this occlusion. Pre-clinical data indicate that therapeutic angiogenesis, the process of administrating exogenous agents to improve and sustain blood flow to limbs, is effective in hind-limb ischemia. Cytokine therapy used for therapeutic angiogenesis currently involves protein-based therapies or gene-based therapies. The proteins delivered are usually via an intra-arterial route and are cytokines aimed at promoting angiogenesis, including vascular endothelial growth factor (VEGF), fibroblast growth factor (FGF), and platelet derived growth factor (PDGF). One study, Therapeutic Angiogenesis with Recombinant Fibroblast Growth Factor-2 for Intermittent Claudication (TRAFFIC), compared two doses of FGF to placebo via catheter delivery in 190 patients with infrainguinal PAD and claudication (9). At 90 days, a single infusion of rFGF-2 was associated with a significant increase in peak walking time compared with placebo (increase of 1.77 versus 0.6 minutes compared to baseline); there was no additional benefit from a second infusion. The pharmaceutical sponsor did not continue with investigation of this cytokine.

The gene-based approaches have involved delivery of "naked" DNA via plasmid or adenoviral gene transfer via intramuscular injection. The Regional Angiogenesis with Vascular Endothelial growth factor (RAVE) trial was the first major randomized study of adenoviral vascular endothelial growth factor (VEGF) gene transfer for the treatment of PAD (10). This phase 2, double-blind, placebo-controlled study was designed to test the efficacy and safety of intramuscular delivery of AdVEGF121, a replication-deficient adenovirus encoding the 121-amino-acid isoform of vascular endothelial growth factor, to the lower extremities of 105 subjects with unilateral PAD. The primary efficacy end point, change in PWT at 12 weeks, did not differ between the placebo (1.8 min), low-dose (1.6 min), and high-dose (1.5 min) groups. Secondary measures, including ankle-brachial index, claudication onset time, and quality-of-life measures, were also similar among groups at 12 and 26 weeks. Of note, AdVEGF121 administration was associated with self-limiting peripheral edema in some subjects. One limitation of adenoviral gene transfer is that re-injection of vector is limited due to immunity. Thus far, none of the above strategies have yielded clinically significant results that would merit FDA approval.

Stem Cells and Claudication

The published strategies using cell-based therapies include a "whole" bone marrow approach versus selective utilization of a specific cell line from the bone marrow or other source, such as vascular or adipose tissue. Thus far, all published therapies utilized adult progenitor cells as there are no published cell-based therapies for PAD using embryonic stem cell lines. Table 8-1 is a partial list of studies using bone marrow mononuclear cells for treatment of claudication. One study conducted by Tateishi-Yuyama et al evaluated the efficacy and safety of autologous implantation of bone marrow-mononuclear cells in patients with ischemic limbs (11). A pilot group of 25 patients with unilateral ischemia were injected with bone marrow mono-nuclear cells into the gastrocnemious of the ischemic limb and received saline in the less ischemic limb. A second group involved recruitment of 22 patients with bilateral leg ischemia who were randomized to injection of bone marrow-mononuclear cells in one leg and peripheral blood-mononuclear cells in the other as a control. The bone marrow aspiration was done using general anesthesia so as to minimize pain and provide for a 500 mL sample. The ankle-brachial index was significantly improved in the legs injected with bone marrow-mononuclear cells compared with those injected with peripheral blood- mononuclear cells ($P < 0.001$). An improvement in transcutaneous oxygen pressure, less pain in pain-free walking time, was also reported and sustained at 24 weeks. The authors concluded that autologous implantation of bone marrow-mononuclear cells is a safe and possibly effective method for therapeutic angiogenesis. This study, although intriguing, is certainly not definitive and requires a larger study with a placebo arm to determine if this strategy is clinically efficacious.

Another strategy of cell-based therapy involves initial mobilization of bone marrow progenitor cells using granulocyte colony stimulating factor (G-CSF) followed by cell harvesting and then subcutaneous injection of the ex vivo expanded cells. Huang et al studied 28 diabetic patients with CLI who were randomized to either cell therapy or control (12). The patients in the cell therapy group received subcutaneous injections of recombinant

Table 8-1.   Treatment of Claudication Using Bone Marrow Mononuclear Cells

First Author	Journal	n	Outcome
Bone Marrow Aspirate Strategy			
Saigawa	Circ 2004	8	↑ TcPO$_2$
Tateishi-Yuyama	Lancet 2002	47	Safe/Effective
Higashi	Circ 2004	7	↑ PFWD, Ach improvement
G-CSF-MNC Strategy			
Huang	Thromb Haemost 2004	5	Safe
Huang	Diabetes Care 2005	28	Pain Improved ↑ ABI
Ishida	Circ Journal 2005	6	↑ MWD, ↑ ABI

human G-CSF (600 μg/day) for 5 days to mobilize stem cells, and their peripheral blood mononuclear cells were collected via cell sorter. These patients then received multiple intramuscular injections into ischemic limbs. Heparin was given as background therapy during G-CSF administration to reduce risk of arterial thrombus. At the end of the 3-month follow-up, lower limb pain and ulcers were significantly improved in the patients of the cell therapy group. Blood flow also seemed to improve as laser Doppler blood perfusion of lower limbs increased and mean ankle-brachial pressure index increased from 0.50± 0.21 to 0.63 ± 0.25 ($P < 0.001$). A total of 14 of 18 limb ulcers (77.8%) of transplanted patients were completely healed after cell transplantation, whereas only 38.9% of limb ulcers (7 of 18) were healed in the control patients ($P < 0.016$ vs. the transplant group). No adverse effects specifically due to cell transplantation were observed, and no lower-limb amputation occurred in the cell therapy patients. In contrast, five control patients had to receive a lower-limb amputation ($P < 0.007$, transplant vs. control group). Angiographic scores were significantly improved in the transplant group when compared with the control group ($P < 0.003$). This relatively small study also does not prove efficacy but suggests that a cell-based strategy may work in patients with CLI. An advantage of using G-CSF to mobilize cells for harvest compared to bone marrow aspiration is a less-invasive approach that provides for larger numbers of cells. There are currently no FDA approved cytokines or cell-based therapies for claudication.

Risks of Angiogenesis

In 1971, Folkman hypothesized that tumor growth and metastasis are dependent on angiogenesis. This concept has generated potentially novel therapies aimed at inhibiting solid tumor growth. This biological effect of tumor growth for angiogenesis raises the specter that therapeutic angiogenesis may stimulate tumor growth in a susceptible individual. Most of the therapeutic angiogenesis studies described above involve short-term stimulation of angiogenesis and not prolonged pro-angiogenic stimuli. To date, none of the studies have reported any significant tumor development, which may take many months for growth to occur. Current studies typically exclude patients at risk for stimulating tumor growth such as those with untreated malignancy or evidence for proliferative retinopathy in the eyes.

There is some concern that therapeutic angiogenesis may promote atherosclerotic plaque growth. Several histopathological studies have demonstrated neovascularization in atherosclerotic plaques in the carotid and coronary arteries, as well as in calcified aortic valves. It is theorized that atherosclerotic plaques use neovascularization as a means to obtain nutritional support similar to solid tumors. The current published clinical studies do not indicate that atheroma expansion occurs to any clinically meaningful level after short-term exposure to angiogenesis-promoting therapies. It is unknown, however, whether prolonged angiogenic stimulation of more than a few months would cause growth of atherosclerotic plaques. One particular cytokine, G-CSF, has been implicated as having a pro-coagulant effect, probably due to increased blood viscosity at the time of induction. This has led investigators who are testing this cytokine to do so with heparin as background therapy so as to mineralize any procoagulant effects.

Considering a Patient for an Angiogenesis Trial

The ACC/AHA (1) and TASC guidelines (13) for PAD both advocate initially a noninvasive medical approach for patients with claudication. The therapy includes risk-factor modification, antiplatelet prescription, supervised exercise rehabilitation, and the addition of claudication medication such as cilostazol. All patients prior to consideration for a clinical trial should receive this optimal care. Patients with lifestyle-limiting claudication who have not achieved a satisfactory improvement in claudication symptoms with medical treatment are potential candidates for angiogenesis therapy.

Studies using cytokine- or cell-based therapy to date appear safe without obvious risk of malignancy increase or progression of atherosclerosis. Interestingly, a placebo effect is commonly seen with claudication studies and ranges from 5%-40% improvement in walking distance on treadmill testing. Therefore, many patients enrolled in these studies may have symptom improvement despite being in the placebo arm of the study. Ultimately only studies with therapy that significantly improves limb perfusion and enhances lifestyle beyond that seen with placebo will be considered efficacious.

REFERENCES

1. **Hirsch AT, Haskal ZJ, Hertzer NR, et al.** ACC/AHA 2005 Practice Guidelines for the management of patients with peripheral arterial disease (lower extremity, renal, mesenteric, and abdominal aortic): a collaborative report from the American Association for Vascular Surgery/Society for Vascular Surgery, Society for Cardiovascular Angiography and Interventions, Society for Vascular Medicine and Biology, Society of Interventional Radiology, and the ACC/AHA Task Force on Practice Guidelines (Writing Committee to Develop Guidelines for the Management of Patients With Peripheral Arterial Disease): endorsed by the American Association of Cardiovascular and Pulmonary Rehabilitation; National Heart, Lung, and Blood Institute; Society for Vascular Nursing; TransAtlantic Inter-Society Consensus; and Vascular Disease Foundation. Circulation. 2006;113:e463-e654.
2. **Khakoo AY, Finkel T.** Endothelial progenitor cells. Ann Rev Med. 2005;56:79-101.
3. **Risau W.** Mechanisms of angiogenesis. NAT. 1997; 386:671-4.
4. **Asahara T, Murohara T, Sullivan A, et al.** Isolation of putative progenitor endothelial cells for angiogenesis. Science. 1997; 275:964-7.

5. Ingram DA, Mead LE, Tanaka H, et al. Identification of a novel hierarchy of endothelial progenitor cells using human peripheral and umbilical cord blood. Blood. 2004;104:2752-60.
6. Hill JM, Zalos G, Halcox JP, et al. Circulating endothelial progenitor cells, vascular function, and cardiovascular risk. N Engl J Med. 2003;348:593-600.
7. Shaffer RG, Greene S, Arshi A, et al. Flow cytometric measurement of circulating endothelial cells: the effect of age and peripheral arterial disease on baseline levels of mature and progenitor populations. Cytometry B Clin Cytom. 2006;70:56-62.
8. Shaffer RG, Greene S, Arshi A, et al. Effect of acute exercise on endothelial progenitor cells in patients with peripheral arterial disease. Vasc Med. 2006;11:219-26.
9. Lederman RJ, Mendelsohn FO, Anderson RD, et al. Therapeutic angiogenesis with recombinant fibroblast growth factor-2 for intermittent claudication (the TRAFFIC study): a randomised trial. Lancet. 2002;359:2053-8.
10. Rajagopalan S, Mohler ER III, Lederman RJ, et al. Regional Angiogenesis With Vascular Endothelial Growth Factor in Peripheral Arterial Disease: A Phase II Randomized, Double-Blind, Controlled Study of Adenoviral Delivery of Vascular Endothelial Growth Factor 121 in Patients With Disabling Intermittent Claudication. Circulation. 2003.
11. Tateishi-Yuyama E, Matsubara H, Murohara T, et al. Therapeutic angiogenesis for patients with limb ischaemia by autologous transplantation of bone-marrow cells: a pilot study and a randomised controlled trial. Lancet. 2002;360:427-35.
12. Huang P, Li S, Han M, Xiao Z, et al. Autologous transplantation of granulocyte colony-stimulating factor-mobilized peripheral blood mononuclear cells improves critical limb ischemia in diabetes. Diabetes Care. 2005;28:2155-60.
13. Dormandy JA, Rutherford RB. Management of peripheral arterial disease (PAD). TASC Working Group. TransAtlantic Inter-Society Concensus (TASC). J Vasc Surg. 2000;31:S1-S296.

KEY REFERENCES

Khakoo AY, Finkel T. Endothelial progenitor cells. Ann Rev Med. 2005;56:79-101. *A complete review of endothelial progenitor cell in vitro studies and clinical studies.*

Asahara T, Murohara T, Sullivan A, et al. Isolation of putative progenitor endothelial cells for angiogenesis. Science. 1997;275:964-7. *The first description of EPCs and function as cells involved in angiogenesis.*

Ingram DA, Mead LE, Tanaka H, et al. Identification of a novel hierarchy of endothelial progenitor cells using human peripheral and umbilical cord blood. Blood. 2004;104:2752-60. *A description of highly proliferative endothelial cells present in the vessel.*

Hill JM, Zalos G, Halcox JP, et al. Circulating endothelial progenitor cells, vascular function, and cardiovascular risk. N Engl J Med. 2003;348:593-600. *A clinical study describing the negative effect of cardiovascular risk factors on EPCs.*

Shaffer RG, Greene S, Arshi A, et al. Flow cytometric measurement of circulating endothelial cells: the effect of age and peripheral arterial disease on baseline levels of mature and progenitor populations. Cytometry B Clin Cytom, 2006;70:56-62. *A clinical method to evaluate simultaneously circulating EPCs and mature endothelial cells.*

Lederman RJ, Mendelsohn FO, Anderson RD, et al. Therapeutic angiogenesis with recombinant fibroblast growth factor-2 for intermittent claudication (the TRAFFIC study): a randomised trial. Lancet. 2002;359:2053-8. *A clinical study of intra-arterial injection of FGF protein in patients with caludication.*

Rajagopalan S, Mohler ER III, Lederman RJ, et al. Regional Angiogenesis With Vascular Endothelial Growth Factor in Peripheral Arterial Disease: A Phase II Randomized, Double-Blind, Controlled Study of Adenoviral Delivery of Vascular Endothelial Growth Factor 121 in Patients With Disabling Intermittent Claudication. Circulation. 2003. *A gene therapy study of intramuscular injection of adenoviral VEGF for treatment of claudication.*

Tateishi-Yuyama E, Matsubara H, Murohara T, et al. Therapeutic angiogenesis for patients with limb ischaemia by autologous transplantation of bone-marrow cells: a pilot study and a randomised controlled trial. Lancet.;360:427-35. *A clinical study of intramuscular injection bone marrow for treatment of caludication.*

Dormandy JA, Rutherford RB. Management of peripheral arterial disease (PAD). TASC Working Group. TransAtlantic Inter-Society Concensus (TASC). J Vasc Surg. 2000;31(1 Pt 2):S1-S296. *International guidelines for treatment of claudication.*

Index